THE
BONE-STRENGTH
Plan

JO TRAVERS

Published by Welbeck Balance.
An imprint of Welbeck Publishing Group Limited
20 Mortimer Street
London W1T 3JW

ISBN 978-1-85906-471-9

A CIP catalogue for this book is available from the British Library.

Printed in Spain

10 9 8 7 6 5 4 3 2 1

This book is not intended as a substitute for the medical advice of
physicians. Always consult your doctor or healthcare professional
in matters relating to health and particularly in regards to any
symptom that may require diagnosis or medical attention

THE
BONE-STRENGTH
Plan

How to improve bone health
for a long, active life

JO TRAVERS

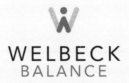

WELBECK
BALANCE

CONTENTS

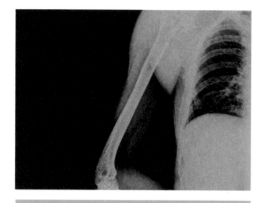

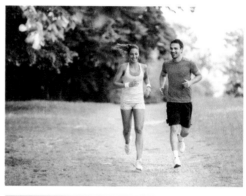

Part 1:

Part 2:

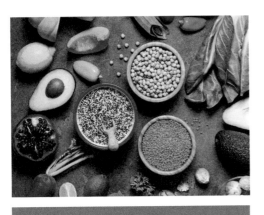

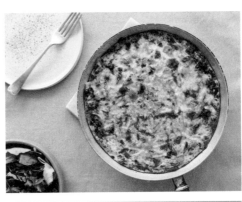

FOREWORD

Good bone health is vitally important to all of us, whether male or female, young or old. We tend not to think about our bones (until we break one!), considering them as inert structures, but as Jo explains in the following pages, they are living tissue that has to be constantly repaired and renewed.

Osteoporosis affects over 200 million women worldwide – 1 in 3 women compared to 1 in 12 men. The maximum amount of bone in the skeleton is achieved soon after linear growth ceases and peak bone density is usually attained by the mid 30s, after which both sexes have a gradual loss of bone with ageing, however major loss occurs in women with decreasing oestrogen at the menopause. Post-menopausal women are the most common sufferers, making bone health of special concern for them, although it can affect younger women, men and very occasionally children.

Rickets is not a problem of the past; it is a condition that affects bone development in children, causing bone pain, poor growth and soft, weak bones that can lead to deformities; adults can experience a similar condition, which is known as osteomalacia. Although the numbers are still small, rickets is increasing in the UK and the most common cause is a lack of vitamin D or calcium.

Exercise, sunshine and a healthy balanced diet are all necessary for bone growth and maintenance. Weight-bearing exercise is excellent, as it allows the entry of calcium into the bones, contributing to improved strength and growth, and the work-out programme in this book is one that is easily followed and incorporated into your daily life. A healthy and balanced diet, from childhood through adult life, is fundamental to bone health to supply all dietary elements vital for tissue renewal and growth. This book has the added bonus of delicious recipes that will help you to maintain bone health.

Vitamin D is essential because it enables calcium and phosphorus to be used to form strong bones and teeth. Sunshine on the skin creates vitamin D; aim for exposure of a reasonable body area for 20 minutes a day from spring to autumn. Vitamin D is also obtained from milk and dairy products, fish liver oils, sardines, herring, salmon and tuna. Jo has encapsulated all these bone facts, and more, in a clear, concise and beautifully illustrated book.

Dr Caroline Marfleet, MBBS, FFSRH

INTRODUCTION

Bones may seem inert, but actually they are very much the opposite: they are constantly changing, growing and remodelling. A good example of how they change over time can be seen if we compare babies with adults. Babies have more bones than adults because some smaller bones fuse together over time. As children grow, their bones also grow with them; and as we age during adulthood, we lose bone mass.

Bones are out of sight, but they shouldn't be out of mind. Worldwide, almost nine million fractures occur every year as a result of osteoporosis alone. Hip fractures are a particular problem, as they often result in chronic pain and mobility issues which can impact independent living. In one study, nearly twenty per cent of people who previously lived in their own home had to move into a care home following a hip fracture.[1] This is where looking after our bones can have a huge impact: reducing the risk of fractures may mean the difference between living out our days independently at home or being institutionalized.

There are some things that we are born with that we can't change. Our genes, for example, have a great bearing on bone health; we also cannot change the fact that we age. There are some factors, however, that we can modify to make a difference to our bones. Bones are complex organs that are affected by our environment, nutrition, medical conditions, medications, exercise, smoking habits, alcohol consumption and more. With all these influences, it can be difficult to know where to start when trying to look after our bones. This book aims to help. Outlining how bones work and what influences bone health, it contains targeted exercises and recipes so that you can start strengthening your bones.

Whoever you are and whatever your age, you need to give your bones some attention – it is never too late to start!

Jo Travers, BSc, RD, MBDA

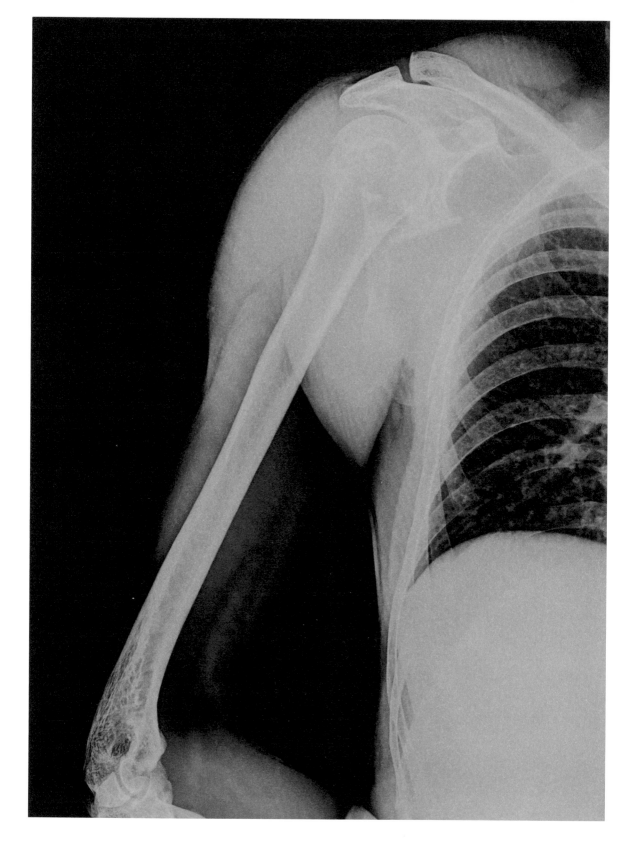

1

THE SCIENCE

Bones play a vital role in the body: at their most basic, they provide structure, protect organs and anchor muscles. In this section, you will learn the science behind bones – what they are composed of, the actions they perform, how they grow and repair, how they are affected by age, lifestyle and hormones, and why conditions such as osteoporosis and arthritis happen and how to prevent them.

BONE BASICS

It could be argued that the primary reason that bones exist is to support the structure of our body, but that's not all they do. Bones work mechanically in combination with muscle to allow us to move, and bone is also protective.

The skull protects the brain, while the ribs provide a defensive cage around the vital organs necessary for life. Bones provide an incredible storage facility for minerals, which the rest of the body can access as needed, and some bones store fat, providing reserves of energy. Bones produce blood cells, including white blood cells, which are an integral part of our immune system, and bone cells also produce some hormones.

The structure of bone

Bones have two distinct layers: a hard, compact outer surface called cortical bone, which makes up most of our bone mass, and a spongy, inner core called cancellous bone. This dual structure fulfils the difficult remit of being hard and strong enough to provide support, but also light enough for us to move around easily, and flexible enough to absorb impact.

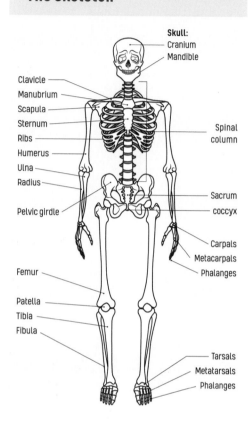

The skeleton

Skull:
Cranium
Mandible
Clavicle
Manubrium
Scapula
Sternum
Ribs
Humerus
Ulna
Radius
Spinal column
Sacrum
coccyx
Pelvic girdle
Carpals
Metacarpals
Phalanges
Femur
Patella
Tibia
Fibula
Tarsals
Metatarsals
Phalanges

Cortical bone

This hard, outer layer is made up of minerals – mainly calcium and phosphate – linked together in a crystalline structure which provides strength. Between each crystal, a nanoscopic layer of a gooey substance called citrate allows the crystals to slide against each other and prevents them fusing together into one large crystal. This structure gives bones their ability to absorb impact and stops them, thankfully, from shattering when we jump up and down.

Bone structure

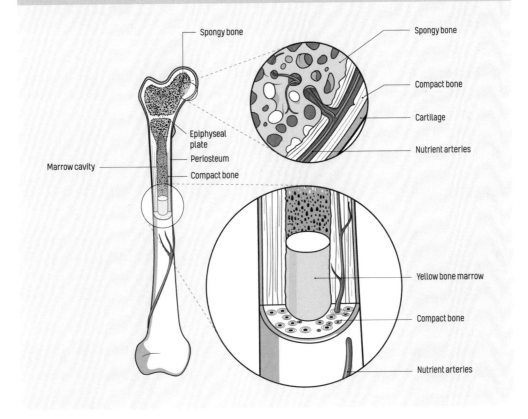

Cancellous bone

This inner layer of porous bone is much less dense than the harder, external cortical layer. It is mainly concentrated at the end of the body's long bones, as well as in the pelvic bones, ribs, skull and vertebrae.

The 'spongy' tissue of cancellous bone is filled with bone marrow, making it the most metabolically active section of bone. This is where red blood cells (that carry oxygen through your body), white blood cells (that fight infection) and platelets (that help blood clot) are

formed. Cells here have a high turnover rate, as they are constantly being broken down while new cells are formed. As we age, much of our bone marrow turns from red to yellow as it shifts from the cell production that fuels growth (red marrow) to a repository for fat cells (yellow marrow). A network of blood vessels connects the marrow to a layer of connective tissue on the outside of the bone, delivering the nutrients and blood that sustain bone growth, health, and healing.

What are bones made of?

The majority of our bone matrix comprises minerals, which are mainly calcium and phosphorus but also smaller amounts of magnesium, potassium, sodium and strontium. The remainder is protein – mainly in the form of a connective tissue called collagen – and water.

Collagen and osteoid

Collagen is the most abundant protein in our bodies; it is the protein that, in combination with mineral crystals, gives bones their strength. Each layer of collagen comprises protein fibres that are arranged in an alternating pattern. These fibres are mixed with a kind of biological 'glue', forming a substance called osteoid. Osteoid helps any newly formed bone bond with the layer beneath. Bone minerals are then deposited in the osteoid, making it hard (a process called ossification).

Cartilage

A connective tissue containing collagen, cartilage joins bones together at joints such as elbows and knees but is also involved in bone formation during the fetal development stage and during childhood. The skeleton of a newborn baby is mostly made up of cartilage, which is gradually replaced by mineral crystals and collagen, forming hard bone. Long bones also continue to grow in

length during childhood through growth plates (known as epiphyseal plates) located at each end of the bone. Bones grow when cartilage cells located in these growth plates divide and multiply, pushing older cells towards the middle of the bone; when these cells die, they are replaced by bone. These growth plates are converted into bone – the epiphyseal line – when a bone has reached its full size, around the end of puberty.

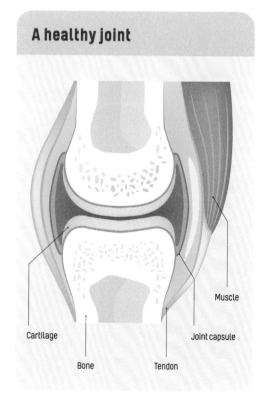

A healthy joint

Cartilage

Bone

Tendon

Muscle

Joint capsule

Cells

Bones contain three main types of cells, each with their own specific function:

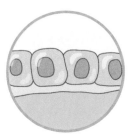

OSTEOBLASTS are the bone builders. They are found on the outside surface of bones and secrete the hormone osteocalcin and also a collagen protein mixture, which mineralizes and hardens to form bone. As osteoblasts secrete collagen, bone is effectively formed around them and they become embedded in the bone. Once surrounded, they become osteocytes (see below).

OSTEOCYTES (literally 'bone cells'), originate as osteoblasts, but once embedded in newly made bone they stop secreting collagen and become communicators. They are integral to maintaining bone health because they tell other cells how to act by releasing chemicals that encourage bone formation or inhibit bone growth. For example, if bones need to increase in strength because you take up running, osteocytes will tell osteoblast cells to start building in response to the increased impact. Conversely, osteocytes will tell osteoclasts (see below) to start dissolving bone and releasing minerals if calcium levels in the blood fall too low.

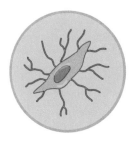

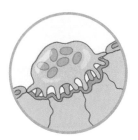

OSTEOCLASTS ('clast' means breaker) secrete enzymes that dissolve and break down bone so that it can be remodelled and repaired. This process releases minerals stored in the bone back into the bloodstream. Like osteoblasts, these cells are found in the compact bone at the bone surface.

Bones are very dynamic organs, which change constantly in response to their environment: they grow, they release minerals and they repair themselves if they get broken. This is all achieved through the actions of bone cells (*see page 13*) in processes known as modelling and remodelling.

Bone modelling and remodelling

Bone modelling is the process of bone growth. This occurs from early on in the womb and continues all the way through childhood and into adolescence. The long bones of the arms and legs grow in length and diameter, and the skull expands in response to the growing brain, eventually fusing its separate plates together around 20 years of age.

Remodelling occurs when existing bone is broken down and new bone is formed in its place. Ten per cent of an adult's bone mass is replaced every year. One reason for this is the replacement and replenishment of old cells. As with all cells in the body, once a bone cell becomes old or damaged and stops functioning properly, it gets taken out of commission. Remodelling can also happen in response to changes in bone use: an increase in weight-bearing activity, for example, will stimulate the production of new bone to cope with increased demand. Conversely, if you stop being physically active, your bone will respond to the decrease in use and discard some of your bone cells.

This process gives us the opportunity to increase bone strength through exercise. However, it is worth remembering that osteoclasts (our bone-breaking cells) work very quickly and can dissolve bone within around ten days. Osteoblasts (our bone-building cells), however, are much slower to multiply, taking around two or three months to fill in the pits left behind by bone-dissolving osteoclasts.

Bone may also remodel in response to the body's need for vital minerals. Bone is a storage pool for phosphate and calcium – vital ingredients in many reactions and body processes. When a need for these minerals arises somewhere in the body, osteoclasts release them from the skeleton and osteoblasts start replacing the used bone.

Remodelling happens in four
distinct phases:

1 Activation

Osteoclasts are activated and new
ones are formed from stem cells.

2 Resorption

Osteoclasts produce acids that digest
bone minerals. Calcium and
phosphate levels in the blood rise.
This process leaves pits in the bone.

3 Formation

As blood mineral levels rise,
osteoblasts are activated and formed
to fill in the pits and make new bone.

4 Resting

Osteoblasts become osteocytes and
resting cells which line the surface of
the newly formed bone.

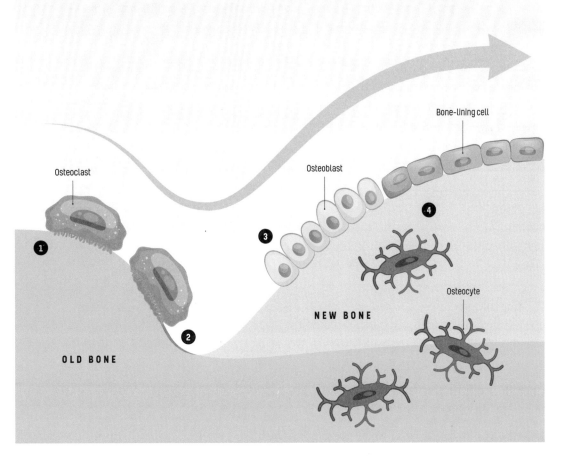

Osteoclast

Osteoblast

Bone-lining cell

Osteocyte

NEW BONE

OLD BONE

Growth and repair throughout life

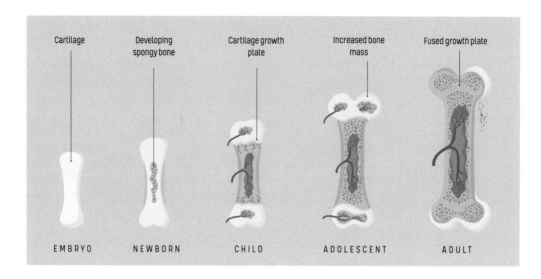

Cartilage | Developing spongy bone | Cartilage growth plate | Increased bone mass | Fused growth plate

EMBRYO   NEWBORN   CHILD   ADOLESCENT   ADULT

Bones are very responsive to our stages of life. In infancy and childhood, they grow rapidly and require a great deal of raw material in the form of calcium and other minerals. Infants absorb around 75 per cent of the calcium they consume, whereas adults absorb only around 30 per cent of the calcium in their diet.

During childhood, long bones, such as those in the legs and arms, have a cartilage growth plate at their ends (see above), which allows them to grow in length easily. When they have reached their full extent in late adolescence, this plate is replaced by solid bone. A similar process happens with the plates that make up the skull, which fuse together in early adulthood when the brain has stopped growing.

Bone mass increases throughout childhood and adolescence as bones grow, reaching peak bone mass (PBM) – the point at which bones are at their most dense – somewhere between the ages of 16 and 35 years. Even after bones have stopped growing, there is a period of time when their mineral density can be increased. In fact, bone building continues throughout life and bone density only declines because the rate of bone breakdown begins to exceed it.

A high PBM is desirable because the higher your PBM, the lower the risk of fractures and bone problems in later life. Attaining a high PBM, however, isn't always a given – some things that influence our PBM can be modified but others, such as our genes, are fixed. Good nutrition during childhood and young adulthood, in particular adequate calcium and vitamin D intake, is a strong predictor of good bone density, while smoking and alcohol use in adulthood can have a negative effect.

Undertaking regular weight-bearing exercise during adolescence can have a massive impact on achievable levels of PBM, as it stimulates bone growth at a time when bones are optimized for growing. Conversely, not making the most of this window for bone growth increases the risk of having weak bones later in life. This window of opportunity closes as we approach our late twenties when the formation rate of new bone starts to slow down.

During pregnancy and breastfeeding, bones are also subject to changes. A growing baby's need for calcium, first in utero and then via breast milk, can cause the mother significant losses in bone mass. This is especially true during breastfeeding, as increased

hormone production during pregnancy gives some protection to bones. Fortunately, once breastfeeding stops, bone loss is largely restored.

Providing nutrient intake is good and plenty of weight-bearing activity is sustained, bone density can remain stable for a number of years in adulthood. For women though, the dramatic reduction in oestrogen production that occurs during the menopause (usually between the ages of 45 and 55) causes significant changes in bone mass. Oestrogen is a hormone that is hugely important for bone health and when depleted causes a rapid loss in bone mineral density of up to ten per cent. This abrupt decline usually occurs in the first five years following the menopause, after which slower, age-related bone loss takes place. Men are only affected by age-related loss, as oestrogen plays much lesser role in male bone health.

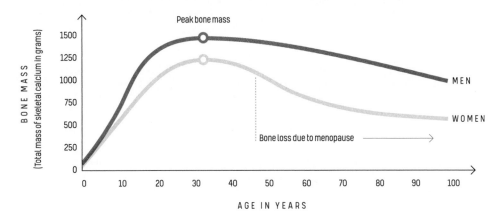

DECREASING BONE MASS WITH AGE IN MEN AND WOMEN

BONE MASS (Total mass of skeletal calcium in grams)

Peak bone mass

MEN

WOMEN

Bone loss due to menopause

AGE IN YEARS

BONES AND HORMONES

THE SCIENCE

Hormones are chemical messengers in the body that effectively tell cells what to do. There are a wide range of hormones that act directly on bone cells, but also hormones that act indirectly through other organs such as the gut and the kidneys, influencing bone metabolism by producing hormones and absorbing minerals. Hormones respond to the environment in the body, so low levels of calcium in the blood will trigger a hormonal response that tells bones to release calcium and the gut to absorb more calcium.

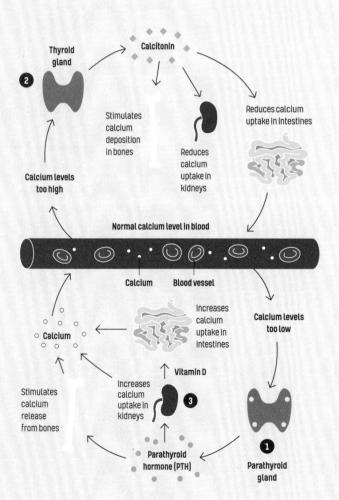

Thyroid gland

Calcitonin

2

Stimulates calcium deposition in bones

Reduces calcium uptake in kidneys

Reduces calcium uptake in intestines

Calcium levels too high

Normal calcium level in blood

Calcium   Blood vessel

Calcium

Increases calcium uptake in intestines

Calcium levels too low

Stimulates calcium release from bones

Increases calcium uptake in kidneys

Vitamin D

3

Parathyroid hormone (PTH)

1

Parathyroid gland

① Parathyroid hormone (parathyroid gland)

Parathyroid hormone (PTH) is produced by the parathyroid gland, which responds to minute changes in calcium levels in the blood. If blood calcium levels are too low, the parathyroid gland increases production of PTH and releases it into the bloodstream. This tells the kidneys to excrete less calcium and tells the gut to absorb more calcium from any food ingested. PTH also stimulates osteoclasts to break down bone in order to release calcium into the blood.

❷ Calcitonin (thyroid gland)

This hormone is produced by the thyroid gland and acts as a counter-balance to the action of PTH. Like PTH, it responds to circulating calcium levels, but is secreted when calcium levels are high. It stimulates osteoblasts to increase bone formation and turns off osteoclasts. It also works on the kidneys and intestines but in the opposite manner to PTH – by increasing the excretion and decreasing the absorption of calcium and phosphate.

❷ Thyroid hormone (thyroid gland)

This hormone helps to deliver energy to cells and works on both osteoblasts and osteoclasts. It is important for bone growth during childhood and regulates bone metabolism in adulthood.

❸ Calcitriol (kidneys)

Calcitriol is an active form of vitamin D that is usually produced by the kidneys. One of its roles is to maintain calcium levels. It stimulates the absorption of calcium and phosphate in the gut and also stimulates osteoclasts to break down bones and release calcium into the body.

Oestrogen and testosterone (ovaries and testes)

Both sex hormones play a major role in increasing bone density during adolescence and early adulthood and maintaining bone mass as we age. Lower levels later in life increase the risk of osteoporosis and fractures.

Oestrogen is produced in the ovaries of women and also in the testes of men. It promotes bone growth and remodelling, communicating with osteoblasts and osteoclasts via oestrogen receptors on these cells. It also reduces bone breakdown by stimulating the thyroid gland to produce calcitonin. Oestrogen can enhance the absorption of calcium by our intestines and reduce excretion by our kidneys to regulate bone growth. Oestrogen production stops after the menopause in women, slowing the production of new bone. Because oestrogen is needed for calcium absorption, low oestrogen levels also result in reduced calcium in the blood, triggering more to be released from bone. A reduction in bone formation is therefore coupled with an increased breakdown of bone, often resulting in osteoporosis. This condition is more common in women because oestrogen levels following menopause are so low.

Research has indicated that testosterone levels in young men are directly linked to bone density. Testosterone stimulates osteoblasts and inhibits the action of bone-breaking osteoclasts, encouraging bone growth and renewal and also the maintenance of PBM in older men. Bone loss in men of a similar age to post-menopausal women is mostly caused by age-related testosterone deficiency.[1] The fracture risk of women is still higher than men, even with this loss of testosterone.[2]

Cortisol (adrenal gland)

Often called the 'stress hormone', cortisol is produced by the adrenal gland and has many actions in the body, including reducing inflammation and controlling blood pressure. It can stimulate bone growth but when levels are too high can have the opposite effect – blocking bone formation and increasing breakdown. Cortisol-type anti-inflammatory steroid medications called glucocorticoids are often prescribed to reduce inflammation and suppress the immune system when treating conditions such as arthritis or allergies, but these can inadvertently cause the side-effect of bone loss.

Insulin (pancreas)

Osteoblasts have insulin receptors, indicating that insulin works directly on this type of cell, although the mechanism of action is not completely understood. Another indicator that insulin plays a role in bone health is that people who have poorly controlled diabetes have an increased risk of fractures.

Leptin (body fat cells)

Leptin is a hormone that increases the number of bone-forming osteoblasts and inhibits the action of osteoclasts. As leptin is released by fat cells, leptin levels are high in people with obesity; it is thought that this is why people with a high body weight tend to have strong bones and lose bone mass more slowly.

Melatonin (pineal gland – brain)

Melatonin is a hormone that regulates our circadian rhythm – the 24-hour cycle that our bodies follow. It is currently being proposed as a novel treatment for osteoporosis because it appears to increase the activity of bone-forming osteoblasts while inhibiting bone breakdown.

Growth hormone and growth factor (pituitary gland – base of brain)

Growth hormone, as its name suggests, plays a role in promoting the growth of all tissues, including bone. It triggers the production of another hormone called growth factor, which in turn stimulates bone growth. In children, particularly during adolescence, these hormones play an important role in bone metabolism, but as we age, growth hormone production reduces and their bone-building action diminishes.

Serotonin (intestines)

A chemical neurotransmitter that acts on brain cells rather than a hormone, serotonin's action on bones is nonetheless similar to hormones like cortisol. Serotonin can both stimulate and inhibit bone growth depending on circulating levels, though quite how and why this is the case is as yet unclear. Several studies have shown an increased risk of bone fractures in people taking medications that increase circulating serotonin levels.[3]

Hormones and bones

The **pituitary gland** is located at the base of the brain and produces the body's **growth hormone** (GH). **Melatonin** is produced in the **pineal gland**, which lies between the two halves of the brain.

The **parathyroid hormone** is produced by the four **parathyroid glands**, located in the neck behind the thyroid. Calcitonin and the thyroid hormone are both secreted by the thyroid gland.

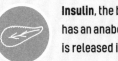

Insulin, the blood sugar regulator, has an anabolic effect on bone and is released in the **pancreas**.

Oestrogen is produced in the **ovaries** of women and also in the testes of men.

Calcitriol, the active form of vitamin D, is produced in the cells of the **kidneys**. **Cortisol** is produced by the **adrenal glands**, located on top of each kidney.

Testosterone is produced by the Leydig cells in the **testes** in men and by the ovaries in women, although small quantities are also produced by the adrenal glands.

Serotonin is found mostly in the **digestive system**, although it is also found in blood platelets and throughout the central nervous system in the **brain**.

(Below the skin) **Leptin** is released from **fat cells** in adipose tissue, sending signals to the hypothalamus in the brain.

FACTORS THAT INFLUENCE BONE HEALTH

We have seen that bone growth and repair are influenced by sex and hormones, but there are other non-modifiable factors too. We are born with our genes and may inherit risk factors from our parents and grandparents for developing bone conditions.

Age also determines bone health as we move from gaining peak bone mass in young adulthood to losing mass in older age. Obviously, we can't stop the ageing clock, but we can do some damage limitation. There are many external factors that influence the health of our bones, and by informing ourselves, we can use them to our advantage.

Weight

One of the biggest modifiable determinants of bone density is body weight. Bone responds to the forces upon it, so skeletons that support more weight need to have stronger bones. This is one instance in which we may see some benefit in having a greater body weight. However, there are several caveats:

greater weight coupled with inactivity is not beneficial to bones; and where weight comprises mainly abdominal fat (especially in adults) there is an increased risk of developing diabetes and other weight-related conditions that can increase the risk of fractures. Several studies have also shown that the quality of bone in people with a high percentage of body fat is lower than in those with more muscle mass, so a higher bone mass doesn't necessarily translate into better bone health.[4,5]

Body mass index (BMI) is a measure of the health of a person's weight in relation to their height. Having a low BMI (low weight in proportion to your height) correlates with low bone mineral density and is a predictor of greater bone loss in later life. Dieting to lose weight – especially by restricting calories – has been shown to reduce bone density and the process of weight loss often results in the loss of bone as well as fat. This is a particular problem for teenage girls who diet: they are already at risk of developing osteoporosis later in life because of their sex and they are impairing bone building during the period when it is most important.

Similarly, women who diet to lose weight during the menopause have been shown to have greater bone loss over a five-year period than women who do not diet. Menopause may therefore be a time when it is best not to try to lose weight.[6] This is of particular relevance because women often gain weight due to the menopause and diet to try to return to their pre-menopausal weight. At the very least, if weight loss is pursued during this time, steps should be taken to minimize the amount of bone lost. Measures might include taking calcium and vitamin D supplements, increasing weight-bearing exercise and getting enough protein to help protect bones during weight loss.

Diet and gut health

The nutrients specific to bone health are discussed in detail in the Nutrition section of this book (*see pages 54–81*), but it is worth noting here that getting the right nutrients at the right time in our lives is essential. A lack of calcium or vitamin D during childhood and adolescence, for instance, will seriously jeopardize bone formation and maintenance. Later in life, lacking these compounds means that we cannot replenish bone tissue effectively.

Diet directly affects the bacterial flora that populate our intestine – our gut microbiome. We have a symbiotic relationship with these 'friendly' bacteria: they feed on the fibre found in the fruit, vegetables and whole grains we consume, and in turn they provide us with essential services. They extract nutrients and minerals such as calcium from food; excrete compounds that directly affect bone cells (stimulating or inhibiting osteoclasts and osteoblasts); synthesize hormones such as oestrogen; provide energy for the colon; train our immune system; and may play a role in reducing stress and maintaining our mental health which can impact bone health.

Gut bacteria, through their relationship with the immune system,

Calculate your BMI

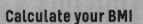

$$BMI = \frac{weight\ in\ kg}{(height\ in\ m)^2}$$

Underweight: less than 18.5

Normal healthy weight: between 18.5 and 24.9

Overweight: between 25 and 29.9

Obese: between 30 and 39.9

Morbidly obese: 40 and above

also play a crucial role in regulating inflammation in the body. This means that disturbances or imbalances in gut flora can stimulate conditions such as inflammatory bowel disease, which can have a significant impact on bone health; conversely, good bacteria (*see probiotics and prebiotics, pages 74–75*) release protective anti-inflammatory compounds into the body.

The microorganisms in our gut are to a small extent genetically determined and this genetic component can influence our base risk for certain bone disorders such as osteoporosis (*see pages 29–31*). However, the majority of our microbiome is determined by modifiable factors.[7] This means we can take positive action to improve the health of our gut biome and to increase its population of beneficial bacteria through diet and exercise.

A lack of calcium or vitamin D during childhood will jeopardize bone formation and maintenance; later in life, this deficiency will affect the ability to replenish bone tissue.

Exercise

Keeping physically active is a key predictor of bone health. As with muscles, there is a very definite 'use-it-or-lose-it' factor with bones. Exercise is one of the most important ways that we can maintain our peak bone mass for longer and preserve bone strength as we age. More information about how bone strength can be improved using exercise, including specific exercises, can be found in the Exercise section (*see pages 36–53*).

Smoking

Smoking harms bones in several ways. It interferes with the action of the hormones calcitonin and oestrogen and encourages the production of high levels of cortisol, leading to bone breakdown and inhibiting bone formation. Toxic tobacco smoke also creates free radicals, which are unstable molecules that can damage cells, including osteoblasts. Smoking damages blood vessels, which leads to interruptions in the supply of nutrients and other substances to bone cells and increases the risk of fractures. Additionally, fractured bones can take longer to heal in smokers compared to non-smokers. But don't let bone health be the only reason you stop smoking – if you are a smoker, giving up is probably the number one thing you can do to improve your all-round health!

Alcohol

Like smoking, heavy alcohol consumption, particularly during adolescence and early adulthood when our bones are trying to establish peak density, can have a detrimental effect on bone health. Alcohol interferes with the production of vitamin D and affects calcium levels, decreasing bone formation and increasing the breakdown of bone, which can lead to osteoporosis. Excessive alcohol use can also disrupt the balance of our hormones, including increasing levels of parathyroid hormone, which pulls calcium from bone, and increasing cortisol levels, which encourages bone breakdown and inhibits bone growth. This has been shown in people with episodic drinking – so-called binge drinking – as well and not just frequent alcohol consumption.[8]

Stress, anxiety and depression

The stress hormone cortisol performs lots of roles in the body. One of its functions is to initiate our fight-or-flight response. From an evolutionary perspective, it is fantastic system: if we were about to be eaten by a sabre-toothed tiger, our nervous system would shut down any immediately unnecessary functions and divert all available energy to either fighting off our attacker or, perhaps more sensibly in some cases, running away. Today, the types of stress we face may have changed, but the system still functions in the same way. Deadline at work? Stress. Money or relationship worries? Stress. Chronic stress is particularly detrimental to bone health because cortisol levels are permanently raised, which means that cortisol is always inhibiting bone formation and exacerbating bone breakdown.

Chronic stress can also tip over into clinical anxiety and depression – conditions linked to low levels of the neurotransmitter serotonin. This becomes problematic for bone health when treatment involves the prescription of a class of antidepressants known as selective serotonin re-uptake inhibitors (SSRIs). These drugs increase levels of serotonin circulating in the brain to improve mood, and there is evidence that high levels of serotonin may inhibit bone renewal.

Other lifestyle factors linked to stress, depression and anxiety, such as poor diet, lack of exercise and alcohol use can also affect bone health.

sleep patterns, have a higher risk of developing osteoporosis and sustaining fractures. Chronic sleep deprivation (for longer than a month) may also affect vitamin D levels, and shift workers may get less sunlight if they work nights and sleep during the day, which can also compound their vitamin D deficiency.

Sleep

Sleep is something we all need in order to function well, but it is particularly relevant to bone health as bone metabolism is linked to our circadian rhythm. Studies have shown that circadian 'clock' genes are present in bone cells. These genes regulate bone remodelling on a 24-hour cycle with osteoblast action peaking at night between midnight and 4am.[9] Not getting enough sleep is associated with a reduction in bone thickness.

Several hormones are also involved with bone turnover during sleep, including melatonin and leptin. Sleep apnoea, a condition in which sleep is disrupted because breathing stops, is a risk factor for osteoporosis, possibly because breathing is necessary (among other things) for our endocrine (hormone) system to function properly. Shift workers, who often have irregular

Medical conditions

The complexity of the systems involved in regulating bone metabolism and the absorption of nutrients means that any medical condition that disrupts these processes can affect bone health.

Hormone disorders

Thyroid hormone (thyroxine) affects the rate of bone replacement, so disorders of the thyroid gland, such as hyperthyroidism (where too much thyroxine circulates in the body), increase the rate at which bone is lost. Likewise, disorders of the parathyroid gland, which releases a hormone that stimulates calcium release from the bones, can decrease bone density and growth. Diabetes, which affects the body's ability to process insulin, and Cushing's syndrome, which causes the over-production of cortisol, also affect bone health.

Disorders of the gut

Conditions that affect the gut, such as coeliac disease, inflammatory bowel disease and cystic fibrosis negatively affect bone health by interfering with the body's ability to absorb nutrients.

Kidney disorders

Kidney failure has a deleterious effect on bone health because the kidneys are unable to properly balance minerals in the body. When kidneys fail, they stop activating vitamin D, which prevents the body from absorbing calcium effectively. Kidney disease can also cause the increased release of parathyroid hormone and a build up of phosphorus as the kidneys stop removing any excess effectively, both of which pull calcium from the bones in an attempt to restore balance.

Eating disorders

Some eating disorders, including anorexia nervosa and bulimia nervosa, are characterized by dietary restriction or purging. This restriction of calories and other nutrients, in combination with a low body weight, is detrimental to bone health. Purging can also affect the body's hormone systems, creating a greatly increased risk of developing osteoporosis early in life. This risk is compounded by a lack of optimum bone mass – many eating disorders arise in adolescence when the body is attempting to, but may be prevented from, achieving peak bone mass (*see pages 16–17*).

Inflammatory conditions

Inflammation in the body presents a range of problems for bone health. Inflammatory disorders that affect joints, such as rheumatoid arthritis, cause bone loss by disrupting the bone remodelling cycle. In these conditions, proteins produced as a result of inflammation cause an imbalance in the bone remodelling cycle by stimulating osteoclast action.

Inflammatory diseases that affect the gut, such as Crohn's disease or ulcerative colitis, have the added complications of reducing the absorption of nutrients necessary for bone health, including calcium, and of reducing calorie intake, which can negatively impact bone growth. Some inflammatory conditions not strictly classed as disorders can also impact bone health. In obesity, fat cells (particularly in the abdomen) emit inflammatory substances, which may explain why obesity can lead to poor bone quality despite the increase in weight-bearing activity. Obesity can also lead to the development of conditions such as type 2 diabetes, which is associated with an increased risk of fractures.

Medications

Many medications affect bone metabolism – some enhancing and some impeding bone growth. Anti-coagulants, such as heparin and warfarin, decrease bone formation and reduce bone density. Similarly, medications commonly prescribed to treat inflammatory disorders, such as glucocorticoids, encourage the death of osteoblasts and stimulate osteoclasts, resulting in a decrease in the formation of new bone and therefore a net loss of bone. Proton pump inhibitors (PPIs), often prescribed to treat acid-related disorders, such as reflux and ulcers, and inflammatory bowel diseases, can also affect bone growth. These drugs work by suppressing the release of stomach acid, but as this acid assists the gut's absorption of calcium, they can prevent the body from absorbing this valuable bone-building nutrient.

When taking these types of drugs, it is particularly important to consider other factors that may mitigate their effects, such as ensuring good nutrition and exercise. Taking the medications in the prescribed manner can also make a difference to bone metabolism. Drugs taken to reduce gastrointestinal inflammation such as omeprazole, for example, are best taken on an empty stomach: ingesting them alongside your breakfast may prevent you from absorbing any calcium from the milk you've put on your cornflakes or in your tea.

There are some medications that are beneficial for bone health and that are used to treat conditions such as osteoporosis. These include bisphosphonates, which regulate bone remodelling, slowing down bone-breaking osteoclasts to give osteoblasts a chance to build new bone. Selective oestrogen receptor modulators (SERMs), which use oestrogen to counter the bone loss caused by decreasing oestrogen levels during menopause, are also protective against osteoporosis. Hormone replacement therapy (HRT) used to be routinely prescribed to protect bones after menopause, but its slight associated risk for cancers and blood clots means that it is not now commonly prescribed for this purpose.

Good nutrition and exercise can help mitigate the effects of medicine that negatively impacts your bone health.

BONE CONDITIONS

Bones are complex organs that depend on nutrients and the right environment to grow, remodel and stay healthy. When a link in this complex chain of processes and interactions is missing, or when conditions are less than favourable, bone disorders can occur.

Osteoporosis and osteopoenia

Osteoporosis is one of the most common bone-related conditions, with 200 million people affected worldwide In the US and UK alone, approximately 30 per cent of post-menopausal women have osteoporosis, with many more having osteopoenia. Both these conditions cause bones to become weaker. Osteopoenia is defined as having lower than normal bone mineral density and can be a marker of progression towards osteoporosis (though it is possible to have osteopoenia and not progress to osteoporosis if action is taken to protect bones). Osteoporosis occurs when bone density drops significantly below that of healthy bone. Diagnosis is made using a bone density scan with bones given a mineral density score. The term osteo (meaning 'bones') porosis (meaning 'porous')

perfectly describes the condition of bones, which feature a honeycomb of large pits and holes compared to dense, healthy bone. This low density weakens bones, leading to the risk of fracture. The bones most commonly affected by osteoporosis are those of the hips, spine, wrists and shoulders.

Causes

Although a family history of osteoporosis is a risk factor for developing the condition, it is not a forgone conclusion. Taking care to modify the factors which can be modified can still prevent – or at least slow down the rate of – bone loss.

Bones are constantly remodelling themselves, but as we age the process of bone breakdown is much faster than bone building, creating the risk that bone density may fall over time. There are two main reasons why this process may tip over into osteoporosis: pre-existing low peak bone mass and conditions that cause bone breakdown.

Developing osteoporosis is much more likely if you already have low peak bone mass. This can occur when insufficient bone is stockpiled during teenage and young adult years – the time when nutrient absorption rates are high and the skeleton is geared up for bone building. Low peak bone mass means that there is

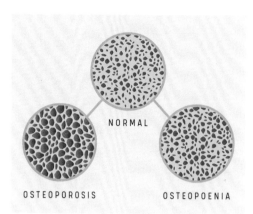

NORMAL

OSTEOPOROSIS   OSTEOPOENIA

maintain the collagen mesh needed to 'trap' the slippery citrate that reduces friction between individual bone crystals deteriorates, allowing citrate to escape. This causes crystals to fuse together and become rigid, rather than sliding over one another, which decreases bones' ability to absorb impacts and makes them more susceptible to fractures.

Symptoms

Osteoporosis is often called a 'silent' disease because it doesn't have many symptoms in its early stages. Fracturing a bone is usually the first indication that someone has osteoporosis: this is particularly common in older women who may experience a relatively minor fall but end up with a serious fracture, such as a broken hip. This type of fracture can severely limit mobility and it is common for people to never fully recover their independence. There can, however, be some visible signs of osteoporosis. Small fractures in the vertebrae can lead to a curved spine and height loss, and are responsible for the condition known as 'dowager's hump', which indicates osteoporosis.

Prevention

There are some risk factors that cannot be modified or changed: these include our age, sex and genetics. Women are much more at risk of developing osteoporosis and osteopenia than men, largely because the menopause causes a

less of a 'buffer zone' for bone loss when osteoblasts are less active in adulthood.

Conditions that cause excessive bone breakdown or insufficient formation of bone can also cause osteoporosis. Inadequate nutrition is a common factor in these conditions. One of the functions of bone is to act as a reservoir for minerals such as calcium and magnesium. When these micronutrients are running low in the body, mechanisms exist to make sure that these elements are released from bone into the blood so that they are available for use.

Other causes include hormone imbalances (occurring in menopause or as a result of hormone disorders), which interfere in the communication between bone cells; a low level of exercise, which means that bone growth isn't stimulated; and a lack of sleep or poor sleep patterns, which can increase the turnover of bone.

As we age, the amount of bone that is laid down by osteoblasts decreases and there are also changes in the mineral structure of our bones. Our ability to rapid decline in bone density. Age also increases the risk of osteoporosis, as bone breakdown begins to exceed bone formation and may reach a critical point. Genetic factors play a role, so that if you have a family history of osteoporosis you are at greater risk.

Happily, there are some risk factors that are modifiable, allowing us to prevent or, at the very least, postpone the development of osteoporosis. Diet is one of the easiest risks to modify (see Nutrition, pages 54–81). If we can get adequate nutrients – especially vitamin D and calcium – through our diet and supplements and maintain a healthy weight (being underweight can cause bone breakdown and prevent bone formation), we can reduce our risk for osteoporosis. Lifestyle factors can also be modified: getting enough exercise (especially weight-bearing exercise) strengthens bones and enhances muscle strength and balance, which can prevent the falls that cause fractures. Smoking and alcohol use are both associated with an increased risk of developing osteoporosis. If you have the luxury of time on your side, making sure you reach a good level of peak bone mass in young adulthood is also preventative.

Treatment

While it isn't possible to cure osteoporosis, there are a number of effective treatments that can slow the rate of bone loss in the disease and therefore reduce the risk of fractures. The most commonly prescribed group of medications that achieve this are bisphosphonates. Other treatments include selective oestrogen receptor modulators (SERMs), which simulate the effect of oestrogen on bone, and occasionally oestrogen hormone replacement therapy and parathyroid hormone treatments, which stimulates the cells that create bone.

Osteoporosis and osteopoenia

Risks
- Existing low peak bone mass
- Poor nutrition
- Hormone imbalances
- Lack of exercise
- Lack of sleep or poor sleep
- Ageing structural changes in the bone and collagen

Symptoms
- Fractures
- Curved spine
- Height loss

Treatments
- Bisphosphonates
- Selective estrogen receptor modulators (SERMS)
- Hormone replacement therapy
- Parathyroid hormone treatment

Arthritis

Arthritis is a condition that affects the joints rather acting directly on bones, but the inflammation associated with the disorder can damage cartilage, leading to wear and friction at the ends of bones. There are two distinct forms of arthritis: rheumatoid arthritis and osteoarthritis.

Causes

Rheumatoid arthritis is an autoimmune condition in which the immune system attacks cells in membranes around joints. These release enzymes that attack cartilage and bone endings, particularly in the hands, wrists and feet.

Osteoarthritis is the most common cause of arthritis and primarily affects the cartilage in joints; it is caused by wear and tear to the joints over time. Risk factors for developing osteo-arthritis include age; the overuse of joints, which may occur through manual labour or in some athletes; being overweight, which puts excess pressure on the joints; and diabetes.

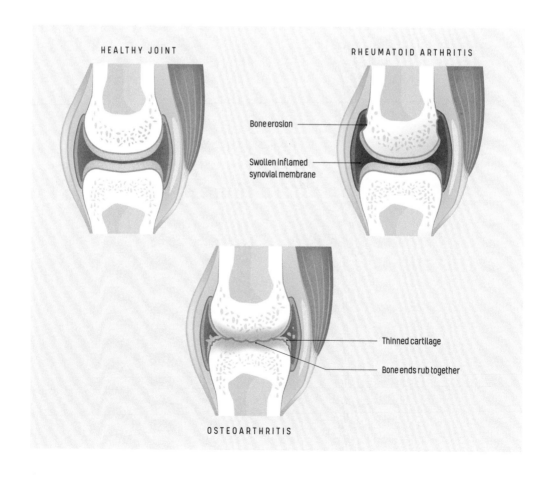

HEALTHY JOINT

RHEUMATOID ARTHRITIS

Bone erosion

Swollen inflamed synovial membrane

Thinned cartilage

Bone ends rub together

OSTEOARTHRITIS

Symptoms

In rheumatoid arthritis, damage to the cartilage and bone endings causes swelling and stiffness in joints, reducing movement, strength and function, which may eventually lead to osteoporosis.

The symptoms of osteoarthritis are very similar to those of rheumatoid arthritis and include pain, swelling and stiffness of joints.

Prevention

As rheumatoid arthritis is a condition of the immune system, it is difficult to prevent. However, people who are older, who smoke and are overweight have a higher risk of developing the condition. Therefore, reducing exposure to inflammatory compounds, such as those found in cigarette smoke, and eating a diet rich in anti-inflammatories, such as fruit, vegetables, whole grains and plant proteins, can reduce the risk of developing the disease, or can improve symptoms. Chronic inflammation also increases the risk of developing other inflammatory conditions, such as heart disease, and has also been linked to depression.

Osteoarthritis can be prevented to some extent by maintaining a healthy weight and minimizing repeated stress on joints.

Treatment

Medication can slow down the progression of rheumatoid arthritis and reduce inflammation, but it cannot cure the condition. The inflammation associated with the disease may be treated with steroids, but this can negatively affect the rate of bone remodelling and increase the risk of also developing osteoporosis by increasing osteoclast activity.

The symptoms of osteoarthritis can be treated with pain and anti-inflammatory medications. Although there is no cure as such, surgery can repair damaged joints.

Osteoarthritis

Risks

- Age
- Obesity
- Mechanical injury to joint
- Overuse of the joint

Symptoms

- Joint pain, swelling or stiffness
- Bony enlargements in small joints
- Pain with cold temperatures
- Crepitus (crackling) in joints

Treatments

- Anti-inflammatory medication
- Joint supports and splints
- Surgery

Osteomalacia and rickets

Osteomalacia differs from osteoporosis because, rather than bone loss, it is characterized by the softening of bones. This happens when newly formed bone isn't properly mineralized – cells lay down collagen fibres but these are not coated with the hard mineral calcium and phosphorous covering that would usually turn them into strong cortical bone. These soft bones may bend or crack. In children, osteomalacia is known as rickets. Common during the nineteenth century, rates have risen again in recent years after nearly a century in decline. People who live in cooler climates, especially if they have darker skin, are at greater risk of developing osteomalacia, as are people who are hospitalized or housebound for long periods of time.

Causes

Most cases of rickets and osteomalacia are caused by a deficiency in vitamin D, which limits the amount of calcium and phosphate that reaches the bones. Sometimes this occurs because of an underlying problem with the kidneys or liver.

Symptoms

Dull, aching pain in the joints and bones, as well as muscle weakness, can be the first indications of osteomalacia and rickets. As the condition progresses, bones may bend or become misshapen, causing bowed legs or a curved spine.

Osteomalacia

Risks

- Vitamin D deficiency
- Diseases such coeliac disease, or kidney and liver disorders, which cause depletion of vitamin D

Symptoms

- Dull, aching pain in lower back, ribs, hips, pelvis and legs
- Muscle weakness
- Bowed legs or a curved spine
- Slower or difficulty in walking

Treatments

- Vitamin D supplements
- Treating any underlying condition

Prevention

As vitamin D deficiency is the main cause of osteomalacia and rickets, ensuring adequate exposure to sunlight, taking vitamin D supplements and following a diet that includes foods naturally high in vitamin D (such as oily fish) or fortified with vitamin D (such as certain cereals and bread) provides the most effective prevention.

Treatment

Most cases of osteomalacia and rickets can be treated with vitamin D supplements. In cases where oestomalacia is caused by another underlying condition, such as a kidney disorder, treating this condition will improve the osteomalacia.

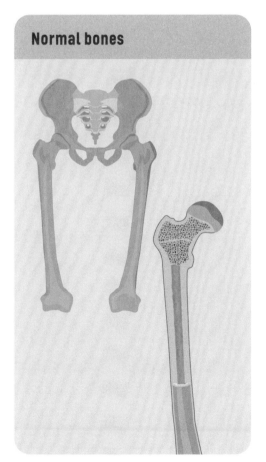

Normal bones

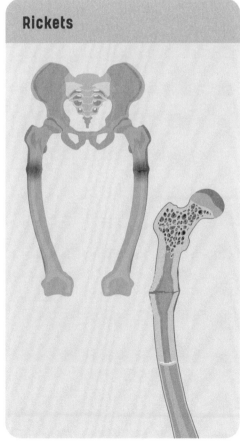

Rickets

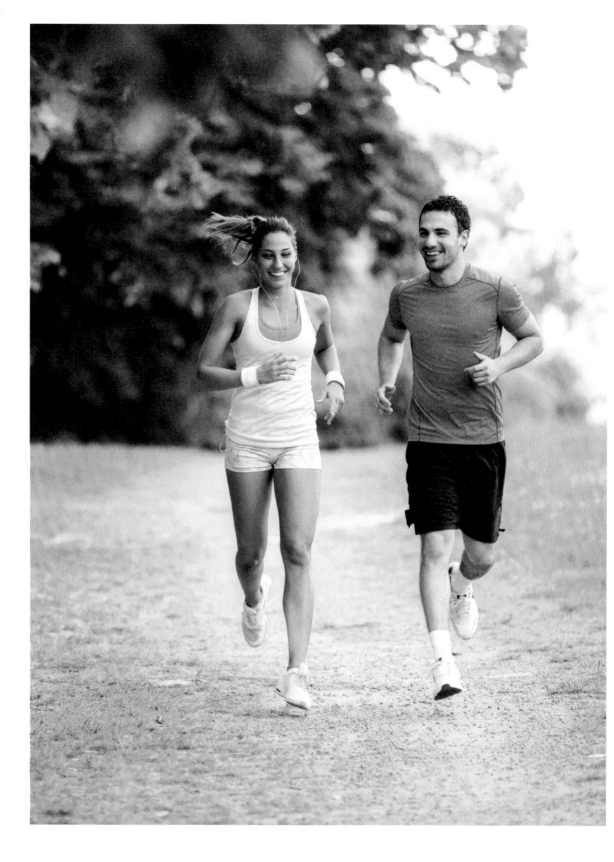

2

EXERCISE

Staying active with the right kind of exercise will help you build bones when young, reduce bone loss as you get older and maintain strong bones to limit the chance of fracture and osteoporosis as you get older. On the following pages, you will discover an easy workout programme for all ages that can be done at home and that provides strength, stability and balance. If you do suffer from a bone condition, you may need to avoid some types of high-impact activity, so always consult your doctor or healthcare provider.

Lifestyle factors play an important role in bone health. We can control many of these factors – choosing to give up smoking, reducing alcohol intake and improving our diet, for instance – all of which have a big impact on whether our bone-building or bone-breaking cells are in action. Arguably the most important lifestyle factor for bone health, however, is exercise, as our physical activity directly affects our bones.

The importance of exercise

The dynamic nature of the skeleton means that it is highly adaptive, reinforcing bones when needed, but also not 'wasting' effort and resources on bones when they are used less. As bones are used, they increase in strength and are better able to resist bone mineral loss and fractures. If we exercise in specific ways, we can strengthen our bones, and if we maintain this exercise level, we effectively maintain the bone – 'locking in' minerals and structural elements. This means that the right exercise can both prevent bone conditions, such as osteoporosis, and help to increase bone density in cases where osteopoenia or osteoporosis have already developed.

Exercise also provides a number of indirect benefits to bone. Improving our physical fitness improves our stability (co-ordination and balance) and our range of movement, which are key to preventing falls and fractures. Exercise can also prevent and improve secondary conditions, such as diabetes, that have an impact on bone health. In type 2 diabetes, a condition associated with an increased risk of fractures, exercise helps to manage blood sugar levels and to burn calories, reducing the body's body fat, which can alleviate symptoms and create a positive cycle that improves diabetes and reduces the risk to bone health.

Benefits of exercise on the bones

- Increases bone strength and resilience against mineral loss and fracture
- Improves stability and balance
- Manages blood sugar levels
- Reduces body fat and increases muscle
- Improves cardiovascular health

Reducing body fat through exercise can also be directly beneficial for bones, because fat cells release inflammatory compounds that encourage osteoclasts to initiate bone breakdown. However, reducing fat is not the same as weight loss – dieting to reduce weight can deprive the body of nutrients necessary for bone building and it does not build muscle strength. Using exercise to build muscle, which weighs more than fat by volume, will help to maintain body weight while reducing body fat; this is much healthier for bones than following a calorie-controlled diet.

Other inflammatory and autoimmune responses that affect bone can also be mitigated by exercise. During exercise, muscles release anti-inflammatory proteins that fight the chronic inflammation associated with disorders, such as arthritis and inflammatory bowel disease, which can impact bone health.

Depression is another condition that is independently associated with bone breakdown and may be improved by regular exercise. Although as yet the mechanisms for this improvement are unclear, they are likely to include the anti-inflammatory effect of exercise.[1] Physical activity also improves cardiovascular health, reducing the risk of heart attacks and stroke, both inflammatory conditions. Not only are osteoporosis and fractures increased in people with these conditions – likely because of associated risk factors – but a patient with heart failure is more likely to die following a fracture than someone without.[2]

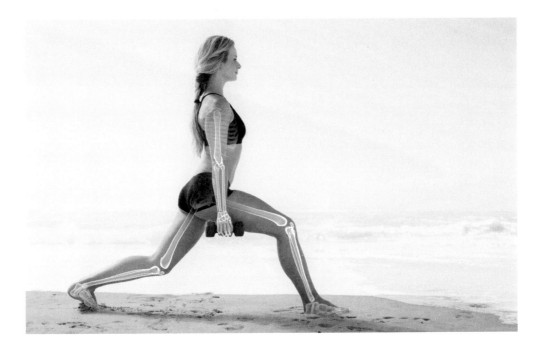

How does bone respond to the forces exerted on it?

Bones are exposed to different forces depending on their type and location. Tension and compression are the main forces acting on bones but long bones, such as those in the legs and arms, are also subject to torsion and bending.

Compression occurs when the weight of our bodies combined with the force of an impact – hitting the ground when we jump or skip, for example – causes bone to compress.

Tension occurs when bone is stretched by the muscles pulling on it. When a bone is bent along its shaft there is compression along one side, while the other side is placed under tensile stress as it bends outwards. This will happen to some extent while lifting weights. In a bicep curl, for example, tension occurs on the inside of the arm and compression will happen on the outside.

Torsion is a twisting force that can happen during a trip or fall, or when we land awkwardly when jumping. This is not the same as straining or twisting an ankle, which refers to damaging a ligament or muscle, but describes the action on the bone itself. A bone can shear if a force is applied directly to the shaft of the bone.

MECHANICAL FORCES ACTING ON BONE

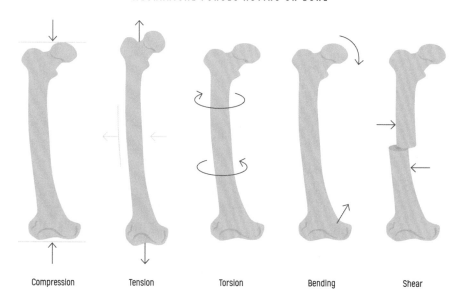

Compression   Tension   Torsion   Bending   Shear

A bone's ability to withstand the stresses exerted on it will determine its resistance to fracture, but too much of any of these forces can cause a bone to break. Bone mineral density and the structural architecture of the collagen fibres in bone determine bone strength and bone can strengthen itself at the sites under the most force through a number of actions.

When bone is under mechanical loading of any kind, this pressure is converted into electrical energy. This energy stimulates the formation of bone cells at the point of stress, followed by the secretion of collagen and bone mineralization. The larger the force – until the point of fracture at least – the greater the bone-building response: whatever doesn't break you, makes you stronger. However, it's not enough to exert force only once – the amount of bone built depends on both the magnitude and the frequency of force. This means that the more regularly you repeat exercise, the stronger your bones becomes.

The opposite occurs – bone strength rapidly diminishes – if you stop using bone. An extreme example of this is when astronauts spend any length of time in space, where the lack of gravity results in a serious reduction in weight bearing. Up to two per cent of bone density may be lost for every month that an astronaut is away. A similar problem occurs if people become bedridden.

Replacing lost bone also takes much longer than the process of losing it, so once an astronaut has returned to Earth, or someone is out of bed, it can take much longer than a month to replenish two per cent of bone density. It is possible, with consistent exercise, to reverse bone loss, but this becomes harder if the period of inactivity extends beyond ten weeks.

Which exercises are best for bone strength?

All exercise, providing it is carried out safely, can confer benefits to health, but improvement in bone health mostly comes from targeted physical activity. Swimming and cycling, which are neither weight-bearing or impact sports, will have significantly less benefit for bones than skipping or boxing, for example. The UK's National Osteoporosis Society recommends some impact exercise most days of the week and undertaking weight-bearing and balance activities on two to three days of the week.

Weight-bearing exercise
This type of exercise includes any activity that involves carrying some weight. Standing, for example, is a type of weight-bearing exercise, because as we hold our body weight up, our bones experience compression through the

downward pull of gravity. To a certain extent, this preserves some bone density – astronauts don't even have this force to help their bones! But standing alone isn't enough to prevent bone loss as we age, and we need to add some extra load bearing to maintain bone health. If we include movement in our load-bearing exercise, such as lifting a weight, we add the force of tension to the force of compression. Movement means that muscles must tense to move bones into position and this increase in force builds both bone and muscle.

Impact exercise

This type of exercise exerts greater levels of compression on bones than simple weight-bearing exercises such as standing or walking. In activities such as jumping, skipping and running, weight bearing occurs as you resist gravity, tension is applied as your muscles work to get you off the ground and, when you land, compression occurs with the force of impact.

Balance and postural exercises

These exercises, which include yoga and Pilates, tend to act more on joints and muscles than directly on bone. However, by helping to build muscle and maintain or improve flexibility (both of which start to decline with age), these exercises improve stability and mobility, decreasing the risk of falls and fractures.

BONE-STRENGTHENING WORKOUT

This ten-exercise circuit training programme is designed to enhance your all-round bone health. The combination of exercises ticks all the key beneficial types of exercise, working with weight bearing, impact, balance and posture to build bone strength and resilience.

By regularly practising this programme, you will build global muscle strength – essential for strong bones – without bulking up. You will also focus on loading the three sites that are most vulnerable to fracture with osteoporosis: the wrists, spine and hips.

Building muscle strength is the emphasis. Stronger muscles pull more on bones and in turn make them stronger. To begin, your body weight alone will provide enough resistance. As you grow stronger, and when you can do two rounds of the circuit comfortably, add weights, and be prepared to keep picking up progressively heavier weights! To increase bone density, it is better to do fewer repetitions lifting a heavier load, than to do numerous repetitions with just a light weight.

The exercises included counteract the classic osteoporotic posture of thoracic kyphosis (forward curvature of the upper back) and excessive chin protrusion. This results in improving your posture through lifting your chest, extending your spine and strengthening your back.

The circuit deliberately does not include exercises with trunk forward flexion, such as sit-ups, and twisting movements, such as the golf swing, which can cause vertebral crush fractures in osteoporosis patients. There are no heavy jumping exercises, as too much high impact can be harmful. Think more in terms of gentle 'spring and bounce' for beneficial bone loading.

Compound, or multi-joint, exercises are included, which make the workout a more efficient way to exercise: you will reap the benefits in a shorter amount of time. The circuit should take 30 minutes from start to finish.

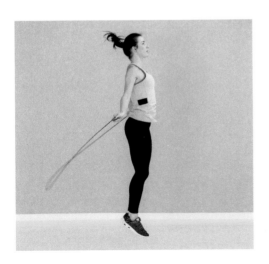

Before you start

If you have diagnosed osteoporosis, check with your doctor that it is safe for you to exercise.

How to do the circuit

- You will need: a mat, a glass of water, dumbbells (optional).
- Warm up for five minutes to mobilize your major joints, such as taking a brisk walk or climb stairs.
- Follow the exercises in order. Perform 8–12 repetitions of each exercise. For alternating side exercises, do up to 12 reps on each side. When you can do 12 easily, it's time to add some weight.
- Allow yourself 15 seconds' rest before moving on to the next exercise.
- When you finish all of the exercises, take a one-minute break – a good opportunity to drink some water.
- Do the entire circuit again.
- Take five minutes at the end to stretch out the major muscle groups.

How often?

Aim to complete this circuit a minimum of two and a maximum of three times a week to reap the benefits. Take at least 24 hours' rest between workout days to allow your muscles to repair and recover. However, on your rest days, make sure you stay active. The circuit will be enhanced if you take other weight-bearing (that is, on your feet) exercise, such as walking, jogging, dancing or tai-chi.

High knees

Simple, yet highly effective, this exercise loads the hips and lower body with the added benefit of single-leg work to ensure each leg works equally. It also helps to improve overall balance and co-ordination.

TOP TIP: To help your balance as you perform the exercise, swing the opposite arm forwards to the knee that is lifted.

1 Stand tall with both feet hip-width apart.

2 Begin marching on the spot, bending elbows to 90 degrees and swinging arms by your side.

3 Pull in your belly button to keep your lower back stable and lift your chest.

4 Start to raise your knees higher – up to waist height if you can.

5 Once you feel confident with your balance, add some bounce through the standing leg.

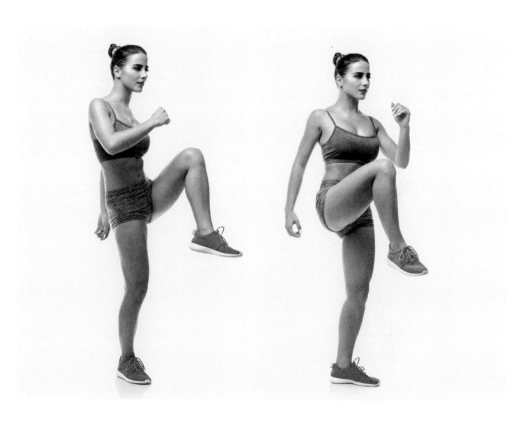

Reciprocal reach

A fantastic exercise for loading your wrists and hips, this also strengthens your core, including important postural back muscles. By moving from four points of contact with the ground to just two, the load increases through individual joints too, which ensures bone density is strong and balanced through all joints.

1 Come into an all-fours position, with your knees under your hips and hands under your shoulders.

2 Find a neutral spine (neither too arched in lower back, nor too flat). Gently pull up through your abs to keep your lower back secure and to stabilize your hips.

3 Slowly reach your left arm out in front of you, extending through your fingertips and parallel to the floor.

4 Lift and extend your right leg behind you in line with your body, keeping your hips level and parallel to the floor. Flex your back foot, pointing your toes towards the ground and push away through your heel.

5 Hold for three seconds, then slowly and with control, draw your arm and leg back into the all-fours position and repeat with the right arm and left leg.

TOP TIP: If you find lifting your arm and the opposite leg makes you wobble, break the exercise down. Lift your arm first, lower, then push the opposite leg away, keeping both hands on the ground. Master this before attempting the full version.

Squat

The squat is a core body-weight exercise that is fundamental to maintaining the strength and flexibility of key muscle groups in your lower body, including your quadriceps (vital for supporting the knee joint) and glutes (hip stabilizers).

1 Stand with your feet shoulder-width apart, toes pointing forwards.

2 Keeping your back straight and your chest lifted, push your bottom backwards and down.

3 Keep the weight in your heels as you sit into the squat and extend your arms in front of you for balance.

TOP TIP: A common error with squats is to bend the knees forwards, when the movement should be focused on your hips. You should always be able to see your toes when you squat, so try imagining there is a chair behind you, just out of reach, to encourage you to push your hips back, rather than your knees forward.

4 Push through your heels to stand up tall, extend fully through your hips, and squeeze your glutes.

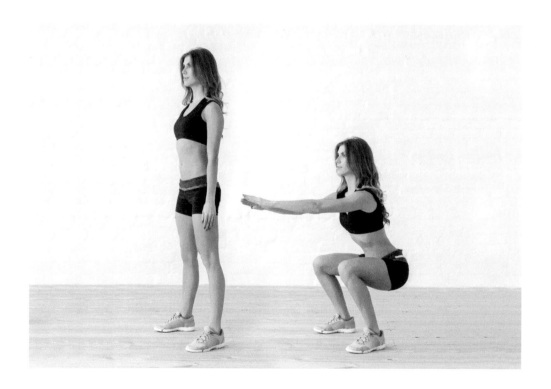

Hand plank

This is a brilliant isometric exercise, which means that you work really hard to keep still and maintain one position! It works your whole body, including the deeper core muscles, as you balance your weight on your toes and hands. Doing this version of the plank (on your hands rather than on your forearms) targets the key wrist area with beneficial bone loading.

1 Start in an all-fours position with your hands under your shoulders and knees under your hips.

2 Pull up your abs and step back onto your toes to extend your legs.

3 Check your bottom is not lifted – you want to maintain a straight line from your shoulders, through your hips and knees, to your heels.

4 Keep breathing as you hold this position for a slow count of 20.

5 To rest at any point, simply lower down onto your knees. Push back up onto your toes when you are ready.

6 To add single-arm loading, try tapping one wrist with the other hand. Progress on to tapping opposite elbows, then opposite shoulders.

TOP TIP: For maximum benefit, squeeze your shoulder blades down and towards your spine, engage your glutes and switch on your quadriceps (thighs). Make sure you continue to breathe through this exercise!

Reverse lunge

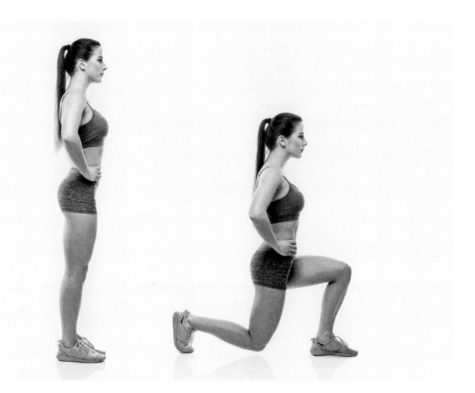

Lunges are an excellent single-leg exercise, testing dynamic balance and leg strength, as well as hip mobility and, crucially, loading the bones in the hips and legs. This version, where you step back instead of forwards into a lunge, is kinder on the knees.

1 Stand tall with your feet hip-width apart and your hands on your hips, elbows gently squeezed back.

2 Step back with your right leg and lower your right knee towards the ground.

3 Push up through your front leg to stand upright and bring your right leg back to the start position.

4 Repeat with your left leg and continue alternating.

TOP TIP: Keep your back straight and chest lifted throughout. If you feel unstable, extend your arms out to your sides for balance.

Superman

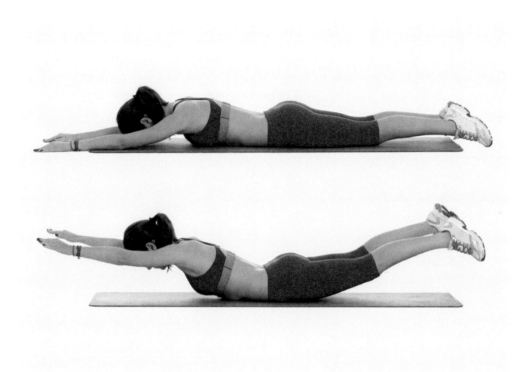

This exercise specifically works the muscles of the posterior chain – the back side of your body. Strengthening the erector spinae muscles is crucial for good posture, combats thoracic kyphosis (forward curvature of the upper back) and brings beneficial compression to the vertebrae.

1 Lie face down with your forehead on your mat and your arms extended in front of you.

2 Pull in your abs, then extend and lift your arms and legs off the mat.

3 As your head lifts, keep your neck long by continuing to look down at the mat.

4 Hold for two seconds, then slowly release down and repeat.

TOP TIP: The lift movement should be small, so don't strain to lift your chest high off the mat. Push your hips into the mat and squeeze your glutes as you lift your arms and legs.

Side steps

This single-leg exercise provides bounce and balanced loading through the hips, knees and ankles, as your body weight is transferred from side to side. It is also great training for your balance because you must engage your core in order to stay upright!

1 Stand with your feet together. Take a step to the side with your right foot and lift and hold your left foot off the ground for one second. Repeat on the other side.

2 Extend your arms out to help with balance, if needed.

3 Next, add some gentle bounce: progress to hopping from side to side.

TOP TIP: When you feel confident, make your steps or hops wider, and keep your free foot off the floor. This increases the challenge and benefit, as the load through the lower body increases and your core has to work harder to stabilize.

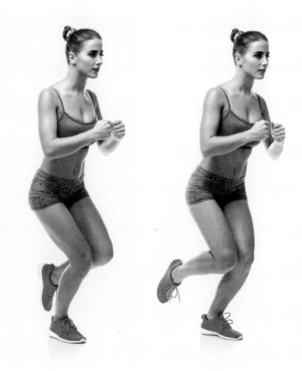

Push-up

This superb full-body strengthening exercise works the shoulder, elbow and wrist joints and addresses mobility, stability and bone loading.

1 Start in an all-fours position with your hands wider than your shoulders and knees under your hips.

2 Step your feet back to extend your legs and come onto your toes.

3 Pull in your belly button to keep your lower back secure.

4 Bend your elbows to lower your body in a straight line towards the floor, keeping your chin tucked in.

5 Push back up through your arms to the start position.

Variation: Knee push-up

If a full push-up is too challenging, start with this version.

1 From an all-fours position, walk your hands forwards and lower your hips to form a straight line from your shoulders to your knees.

2 Pull in your belly button, then bend your elbows to lower your chest and hips towards the floor, keeping your chin tucked in.

3 Push back up through your arms to the start position.

> **TOP TIP:** It's a good idea to practise a mix of knee and full push-ups. It's important to build strength by trying the full version, even if you can only manage a few repetitions with a limited range.

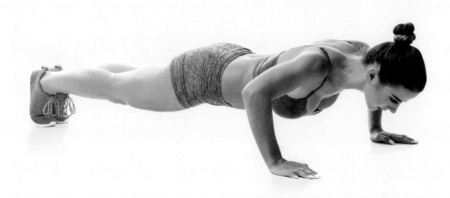

Deadlift

This is the go-to exercise for working your posterior chain. Technique is important, as the deadlift targets your erector spinae (for upright posture), hamstrings and glutes. Strengthening all of these muscles will provide more resistance and improve bone density in your spine and hips.

1 Pick up a weight (two dumbbells or food tins).

2 Stand tall with your feet hip-width apart, knees soft and hold your weights alongside your thighs.

3 Draw your shoulder blades back and down, roll your weight into your heels, then hinge forward from your hips, keeping your spine neutral, slowly lowering the weights to knee level.

4 Make sure you keep your back straight and don't slump forward.

5 To return to standing, lift your chest and fully extend through your hips.

TOP TIP: Notice that in a deadlift you don't sink your hips low as you do in a squat. You can do this without weights: place your hands on your thighs, then slide your fingertips down the front of your thighs to just below your knees as you bend.

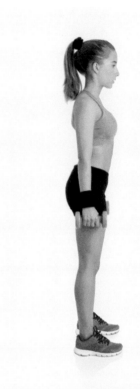

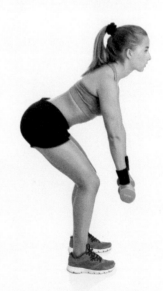

Side lunge

The side-to-side movement in this exercise provides beneficial compression to the hips from a side angle. It also strengthens the major muscles around the hips, which helps with global stability in the body.

1 Start with your feet together, toes facing forward.

2 Take a big step out to the side with your right leg, bend the knee and push the hips backwards to sink into the side lunge. Keep your left leg straight.

3 Push off your right leg to come back up to standing with your feet together.

4 Repeat with your left leg and continue alternating.

5 Gradually increase the width of your step and the depth of your lunge.

TOP TIP: Look straight ahead of you, not down at the ground, when performing the side lunge. This will help you to keep your back straight and chest lifted.

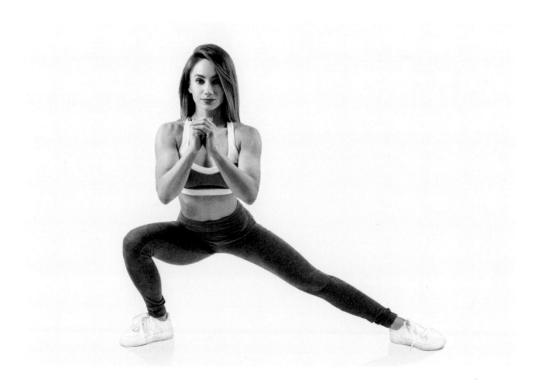

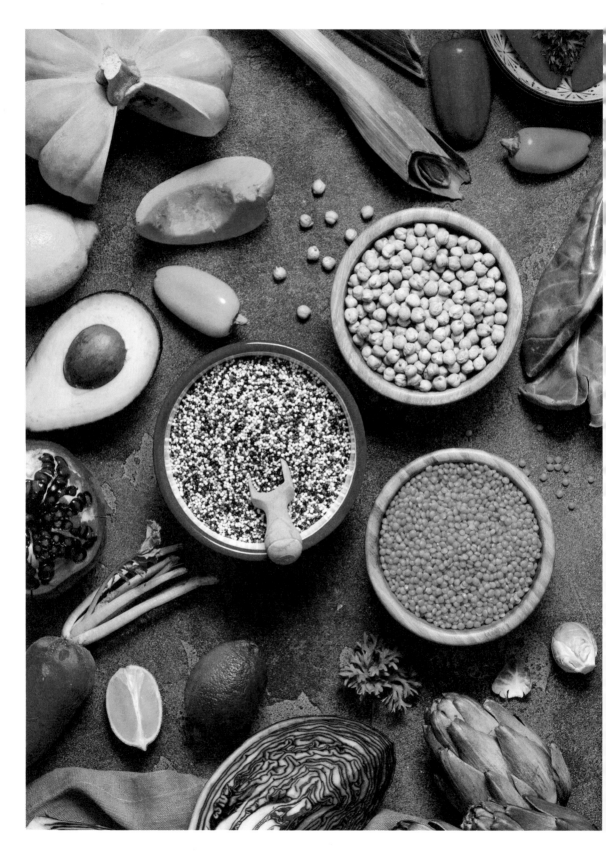

NUTRITION

By understanding the key nutrients, minerals and compounds you need for bone health – what they do, where you can get them and daily recommendations – you can actively include them in your diet to increase your body's ability to repair and maintain your bones. Along with protein, calcium, iron, zinc and a host of others, you will discover the role of phytonutrients, prebiotics and probiotics, as well as which compounds to avoid, and which diets impact bone health.

WHY DOES NUTRITION MATTER?

NUTRITION

The old adage 'you are what you eat' is particularly applicable to bone because of the delicate interplay of nutrients involved in creating and activating bones cells. The formation of osteoblasts and osteoclasts from stem cells, and their activity and maintenance, depend on complex processes that use vitamins and minerals as catalysts and co-factors. The structural elements of bone – the proteins and minerals that fuel the processes of mineralization and ossification – are also derived from diet.

As well as providing the ingredients that make up bone and fuelling the processes that form bone, compounds in our diet regulate inflammation in the body, which can affect bone turnover. The digestion of saturated fats, for example, produces an inflammatory response

that has a negative effect on bone, while fruit and vegetables produce anti-inflammatory compounds, which protect against conditions that adversely affect bone health.

In looking at the nutrients most helpful for bone health, it is important to consider special diets and supplements, many of which claim to solve a variety of problems, but not all have a positive impact on bones, and some may even be detrimental. Restricting calories may achieve weight loss, for example, but is not necessarily good for bone health.

By understanding what constitutes a healthy diet for bones, however, we can take positive action to fuel bone formation, maintenance and ongoing strength through what we choose to eat, and can also protect ourselves from developing other conditions that negatively impact our bones.

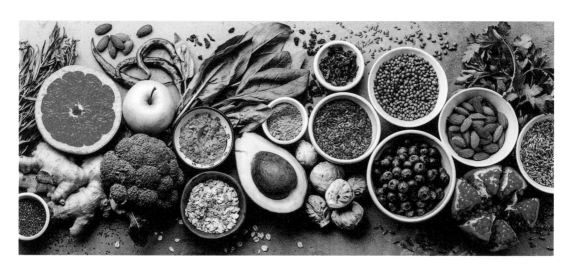

Bones need energy

Some reactions that occur in the body don't require energy to fuel them, but the processes linked to bone are very energy dependent. Bone requires energy to, among other things, activate vitamin D, absorb calcium and create osteoblasts from stem cells. This energy is provided by the food and drink we consume and the nutrients that these contain.

In basic terms, energy is measured in calories and a calorie is defined as the amount of energy it takes to raise the temperature of water by one degree. It can be difficult to extrapolate this to the number of calories in a biscuit, but it does give us an idea of how food contributes to our overall energy needs. Most foods contain some energy, but the best sources are carbohydrates (3.75 kcal per gram), protein (4 kcal per gram) and fat (9 kcal per gram).

It is estimated that women need around 2,000 kcals per day and men 2,500 kcals, but in practice it is a bit more complicated than that. Calorie requirements are dependent on how much activity (or inactivity) is undertaken and our metabolic rate. In clinic, as a rough guide, I prefer to use 30 kcals per kilogram of body weight to estimate requirements, rather than the generic daily average. If you are a woman weighing 60 kilograms, this

gives a daily estimated requirement of 1,800 kcal (if you then consumed the generic average amount of 2,000 kcal per day, you would probably gain weight over time). A man weighing 100 kilograms would need closer to 3,000 kcal per day in order to cover his metabolic requirements and activity.

Having enough energy available to fuel bone remodelling is vital for maintaining bone density and strength. Calorie-controlled diets that restrict nutrients and poor diets that do not contain a good balance of high-quality nutrients can both affect the energy available to bones. Exercising (which depletes energy) in combination with restricting calories can be particularly detrimental to bone health, especially in older women following menopause who have diminished bone density.

Having enough energy available to fuel bone remodelling is vital for maintaining bone density and strength.

NUTRITION

Protein

Protein is a key nutrient requirement for strong bones because, along with calcium and phosphorus, it makes up a significant part of the bone matrix. As bones are continually remodelled, this nutrient is in constant demand and so we need a regular supply.

How it works

The proteins we eat are digested and broken down into their constituent parts, called amino acids. These amino acids are then reassembled into new protein structures used throughout the body – in the case of bones, they primarily form collagen.

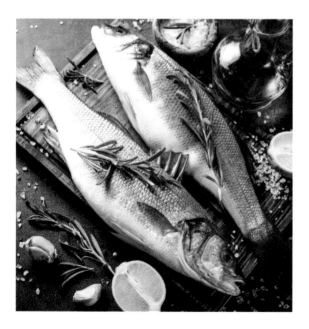

Sources

Although proteins are found in almost all foods, the main dietary sources are meat, fish, eggs, dairy, beans and nuts.

Requirements

The recommendations for the average protein intake per day for adults are 0.8 grams per kilogram of body weight. This means that if you weigh 60 kilograms you will need around 48 grams of protein per day. To give this some context, an egg contains around 17 grams, 100 grams of red kidney beans contains about 9 grams, and a 120-gram chicken breast contains about 37 grams. There is no evidence to suggest that either meat or plant proteins are better for bones, but animal-derived proteins do tend to contain more protein per gram than plant-based sources. So if you are a vegetarian or vegan, you may have to try a bit harder to get what you need.

There is evidence to suggest that older adults may need more protein to maintain bone density. Some studies have suggested that they need 0.84 grams per kilogram body weight per day.

Children also need considerably more protein per kilogram of body weight to support growth. This is especially important during adolescence when the body is trying to achieve peak bone mass.

Calcium

Calcium is a 'macro' mineral, meaning that we need a lot of it compared to some other minerals. It makes up 1.5–2 per cent of our total body weight, which may not sound like much, but compared to other minerals such as boron – which contributes less than 10 milligrams – it is a fairly significant quantity.

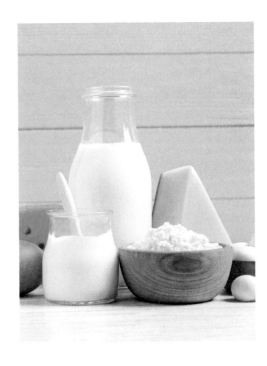

How it works

Most of the calcium in our body (99 per cent) is found in bones and teeth and, in combination with collagen and phosphorus, it makes bones hard. Bones also act as a calcium reservoir, supplying this nutrient to fuel metabolic processes elsewhere in the body. Calcium cannot be absorbed in large enough quantities to build bone without vitamin D. This is because vitamin D plays a key role in the synthesis of a protein that allows calcium to pass through the gut wall. Without this calcium-binding protein, calcium stays in the digestive tract and is excreted rather than absorbed.

Calcium's interdependence on vitamin D makes it difficult to assess its levels and actions in isolation. The body ensures that blood calcium levels remain stable by immediately initiating the release of calcium from bones into the bloodstream when needed, so a blood test isn't the best way to assess – a bone scan is much more effective.

Sources

The best-known source of calcium is, of course, dairy products, but it can also be found in the bones of tinned fish, kale and broccoli, beans and lentils, dried fruit and fortified products such as milk alternatives and breakfast cereals. It is worth noting that calcium tends to be better absorbed from dairy sources because lactose (the sugar present in milk) enhances absorption. Calcium in fortified milk alternatives falls as a sediment to the bottom of the carton, so even when fortified at the same level as dairy, a glass of soy milk may not provide anywhere near the same quantity of calcium as a glass of dairy milk.

Calcium often binds to other molecules and minerals when it is eaten with other foods.[1] If these compounds are not easily absorbed, then the calcium will also be lost. Phytates (found in whole grains) and oxalates (found in spinach and berries) are examples of such compounds. Some animal studies have shown that intestinal bacteria such as bifidobacterium, found in fermented foods like yogurt and sauerkraut, seem to be able to reduce the binding of calcium to phytates and oxalates by converting fibre to short chain fatty acids. The acidic nature of these compounds also enhances calcium absorption.

Zinc and magnesium can also affect circulating calcium levels, as they compete with calcium for absorption and can therefore block some calcium from getting through the absorption pathways from the gut. Caffeine and sodium increase the amount of calcium that is excreted in the urine so it is advisable to moderate intake of salt and caffeine.

Requirements

We need around 700 milligrams of calcium per day and a 250-millilitre glass of milk contains almost half of this.

Good sources of calcium

- Milk, cheese and other dairy foods
- Green leafy vegetables, such as broccoli, cabbage and okra, but not spinach
- Soya beans
- Tofu
- Soy drinks with added calcium
- Nuts
- Bread and anything made with fortified flour
- Fish where you eat the bones, such as sardines and pilchards

For vegans:
- Fortified soy, rice and oat drinks
- Calcium-set tofu
- Sesame seeds and tahini
- Pulses
- Brown and white bread (with calcium added)
- Dried fruit such as raisins, prunes, figs and apricots

Vitamin D

Vitamin D is a vital nutrient for bone health, but it isn't really a vitamin in the true sense of the word because it functions like a hormone. A vitamin is usually defined as a nutrient that is essential for body function but that cannot be made by the body, so must be taken through our diet. Vitamin D is essential, but our body can manufacture it, and it is actually found in very few foods. We usually produce vitamin D in our skin in the presence of sunlight. It must be 'activated' before it can perform its functions, and this activation changes it to a hormone called calcitriol, which then acts on cells.

How it works

Vitamin D receptors are found in a range of cells throughout the body and affect many processes, including the regulation of brain chemicals, supporting the immune system and bone mineralization. Some functions are possibly still unknown, but its role in bone health has been well understood since the early twentieth century when it was discovered that vitamin D deficiency was the primary cause of rickets. Deficiency also plays a role in osteomalacia, osteopoenia and osteoporosis.

When the parathyroid gland detects that calcium levels in the blood are low, it releases parathyroid hormone to stimulate vitamin D activation. Once activated, vitamin D increases absorption of phosphorus and calcium in the intestine, but also stimulates osteoclasts to release minerals from bone into the bloodstream.

Sources

Most vitamin D is made in the skin, but this can only occur with enough exposure to sunlight. Dietary sources include liver, eggs, oily fish, butter, fortified foods such as yogurt and cereals, and of course supplements.

Vitamin D is fat-soluble, meaning that it does not dissolve in water and is best absorbed by the bloodstream alongside fat. This means that if you are taking a supplement it is a good idea to take it with a meal containing some fat.

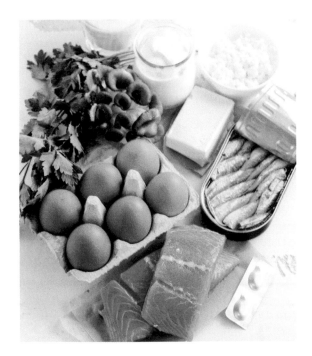

Requirements

The recommended vitamin D intake is 10 micrograms per day. In some northern European countries, such as the UK and Denmark, the current advice is that most people should be able to make enough vitamin D between April and September, but during winter months, when sunlight in northern Europe is not strong enough to trigger synthesis, a supplement is suggested for those populations that don't get the recommended 10 micrograms from other sources.[2]

For some adults, such as those with darker skin or those who don't go outside much or cover their skin with clothes or sun cream, it may be necessary to take a vitamin D supplement all year round. Vitamin D deficiency has been found to be more prevalent in the Middle East than in northern Europe despite the differences in sunlight availability, most likely due to people spending less time actually in the sun.[3]

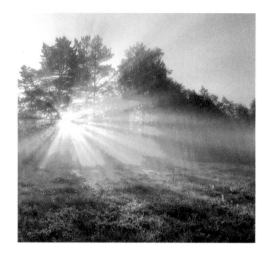

During winter months, when sunlight in northern Europe is not strong enough to trigger synthesis, a supplement is suggested for those populations that don't get the recommended 10 micrograms.

Good sources of vitamin D

- Oily fish, such as salmon, sardines and mackerel
- Eggs
- Fortified fat spreads
- Fortified breakfast cereals
- Some powdered milks

For vegans:
- Sunlight
- Vitamin D supplements
- Fat spreads, breakfast cereals and soy drinks with vitamin D added

Phosphorus

Phosphorus is the second most abundant mineral in the body (making up one per cent of our total body weight) and, with calcium, is the major structural component of bone and teeth. It also plays other roles in the body, balancing pH levels in the blood, helping with cell repair and helping to turn fat, carbohydrates and protein into energy.

How it works

Phosphorus is mainly found in the bones in the form of phosphate, which joins with calcium to make bone's strong crystalline structure. For this process to work effectively, and for phosphorus to fulfil its other roles in the body, it is extremely important that calcium and phosphate levels in the bloodstream are balanced. Like calcium, the absorption of phosphate is regulated by vitamin D,

and blood levels are controlled by parathyroid hormone and the hormone calcitonin. Parathyroid hormone stimulates the release of phosphate and calcium from the bones and from the gut when bloodstream levels need to rise; calcitonin prevents osteoclasts breaking down bone (encouraging bone mineralization) and stimulates the kidneys to excrete phosphate in the urine when blood levels need to fall.

Sources

Phosphorus is found in a wide variety of foods but is most abundant in those with high levels of protein, such as meat, fish, eggs and dairy products. Phosphorus is also present in nuts, seeds, beans and whole grains, in the form of phytate. Phosphate is bound to carbon hydrogen and oxygen.

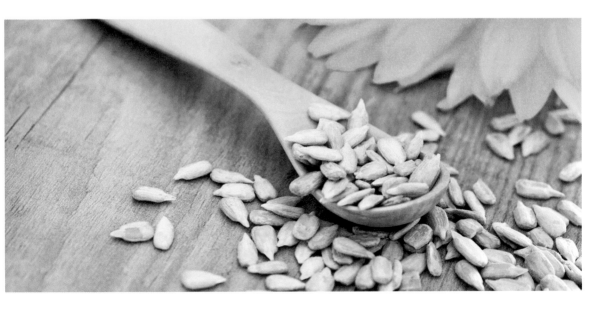

Phosphate in this form is less well absorbed by the body because it is bound into the molecule, but may be accessed more readily by consuming sprouted seeds and beans or fermented foods such as the fermented soy product tempeh.

Requirements

Adults require 550 milligrams of phosphorus daily, which is generally easy to achieve: an 85-gram portion of meat or fish will provide about a third of this and a 30-gram serving of cheese will provide around a quarter. Tempeh contains around half of the daily requirements per 100 grams. As so many foods contain phosphorus, most people get the amount they need through their diet, but excessive alcohol use, some medications (especially antacids containing calcium and magnesium which bind with phosphate and prevent absorption), and diabetes may cause levels to drop too low. Excess consumption can also be harmful, especially in people with kidney disease, who may find it difficult to clear phosphorus from their blood. Phosphate's relationship with calcium means that high levels can lead to processes that pull calcium out of bones, impacting bone health, and can also lead to dangerous calcium deposits in blood vessels and other body tissues.

Zinc

Zinc is an essential mineral needed for many body processes including immune system function, protein synthesis and the action of many enzymes including some that are specific to bone health.

How it works

Zinc helps to change stem cells into different types of bone cells and also plays a role in bone metabolism. It helps to generate the collagen protein matrix on which calcium and phosphate are deposited when bone is formed, and helps in the repair and remodelling of bone by suppressing the formation of osteoclasts, stimulating the death of mature osteoclasts and promoting osteoblast action (*see also bone remodelling, pages 14–15*). Zinc is needed for calcium absorption and low levels are associated with a risk of osteoporosis. The effects of zinc deficiency on bone can be seen clearly in children where it impairs cartilage and collagen production, retarding growth. As well as sustaining bone health, zinc affects the enzymes in our digestive system – low levels reduce the enzymes necessary for extracting protein from food for use in our bodies.

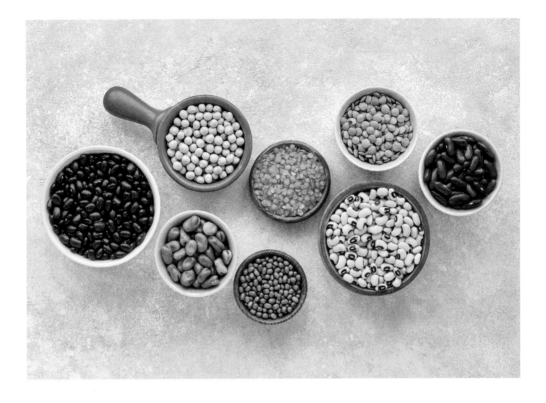

Sources

Zinc is found mainly in foods with a high protein content, such as meat and fish, but also in legumes, nuts, cereals and some vegetables, including mushrooms, kale and spinach. For vegetarians and vegans, beans can be an important source of zinc, although absorption of the mineral is inhibited by phytates which are also found in beans. Vitamin C may aid in the absorption process, so although fruit and vegetables aren't the best sources of zinc, eating a good variety can contribute to overall zinc absorption.

As with calcium, zinc is more readily absorbed in an acidic environment, so taking medications such as proton pump inhibitors, which reduce the production of stomach acid, and antacids that create an alkaline environment can block absorption.

Requirements

To ensure sufficient zinc levels, 9.5 milligrams per day is recommended for men and 7 milligrams per day for women. Teenage girls and boys require 9 milligrams per day and not getting this amount is very likely to affect peak bone mass. A serving of 80 grams of minced beef contains around 3.8 milligrams, 250 millilitres of milk provides 0.5–o 1.2 milligrams, but interestingly, a single oyster will give you around 13 milligrams!

Magnesium

Found in all body cells, magnesium is a mineral that helps with many biochemical processes; these include maintaining nerve and muscle function, metabolizing energy and especially the regulation of bone strength. Sixty per cent of the magnesium in our body is located in our bones, a third of this on the surface of bones in the cortical layer, which acts as a reservoir, releasing magnesium into the bloodstream as needed; the remaining two-thirds forms the crystal structure of bone along with calcium and phosphorus.

How it works

In addition to its role in hundreds of chemical reactions, magnesium is needed to activate vitamin D, to form new calcium crystals and to regulate the absorption and release of calcium from bones, all of which influence bone remodelling. Magnesium deficiency is therefore a strong risk factor for developing osteoporosis and, conversely, adequate magnesium intake in childhood has been shown to be a predictor for high bone mineral density in later life.

There is still much that is unknown about magnesium, especially in relation to bone health, but it does seem that the beneficial effects of magnesium on bone can be reversed if levels are too high, either through kidney disease or excessive supplements. Calcium and magnesium share the same absorption pathways, so one can block absorption of the other.

Having excessive magnesium in the blood may interfere with bone mineralization as the excess becomes joined in bone with phosphorus as magnesium phosphate – meaning less phosphorus is available to join with calcium to make bone-forming calcium phosphate. High intakes may also affect the regulation of parathyroid hormone.

Sources

Nuts, seeds, beans (including coffee and cocoa) and legumes, green leafy vegetables and whole grains are all good sources of magnesium.

Requirements

Daily intake of magnesium is needed to ensure that bone stores are not depleted. Men need 300 milligrams per day and women need 270 milligrams per day. Teenagers of either sex need 300 milligrams per day. A cup of cooked spinach provides about 150 milligrams and one tablespoon of pumpkin seeds provides about 75 milligrams. A double shot of espresso will give you around 50 milligrams.

Copper

Copper, like zinc, is a mineral that is necessary for some vital enzyme functions related to bone health. Although there is still a lot to be learned about copper's role in the bones, we know that copper deficiency leads to bone malformation.

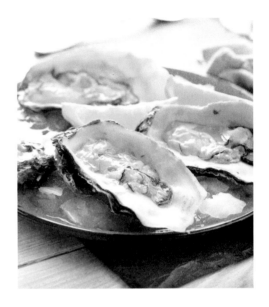

How it works

One of copper's enzymatic jobs appears to be helping to produce collagen and increasing the strength of bone matrix; it is also thought to aid the formation of osteoblasts from stem cells. Copper has been shown to be beneficial for the success of bone grafts, too, as it encourages bone to regrow and has antibacterial properties.

Copper is a co-factor in the production of various antioxidants. One of these copper-dependent compounds inhibits bone breakdown by neutralizing the free radicals used by osteoclasts to dissolve bone. Copper deficiency therefore negatively affects bone mineral density, but too much copper has also been found in a recent study to increase the risk of fractures, indicating that a fine balance is needed. Copper toxicity can cause kidney damage, which given the kidneys' role in bone health, might be the reason for its association with higher fracture risk.

Sources

Liver, oysters, lobster, beans, nuts and potatoes are all dietary sources of copper. Copper absorption in the intestine is enhanced by an acidic environment and vitamin C (itself an acid) also aids in the absorption. Antacids that create an alkaline environment and PPI (proton pump inhibitor) medication that blocks acid production in the stomach can reduce absorption rates.

Requirements

We don't need much copper, just 1.2 milligrams per day, which should be easy to get from a varied and balanced diet.

Fluoride

Fluoride is a mineral that contributes to the mineralization of bones and the formation of tooth enamel.

How it works

In bones, fluoride stimulates the production of osteoblast cells; in teeth, it acts on the cells that form and then protect tooth enamel.

Sources

Fluoride in the diet mainly comes from water, but its levels are dependent on geography. In some areas where naturally occurring levels are low, drinking water is fortified with fluoride as a means of protecting teeth from decay.

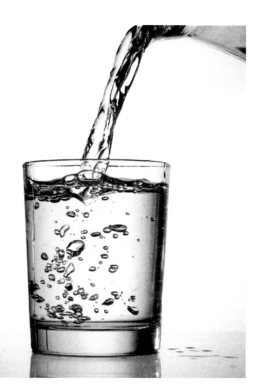

Another source of fluoride is toothpaste, which contributes to fluoride intake if swallowed. This has been shown to increase the risk of fluorosis in teeth (staining, surface irregularities and pitting), but also less frequently in bones, from excessive toothpaste use over time. Ensuring that young children do not swallow toothpaste, particularly in the first eight years when adult teeth are developing, can protect teeth from discolouration.

Requirements

Fluoride is a naturally occurring compound, but the levels necessary for health are still debated. While there is evidence that adding fluoride to public water supplies can reduce teeth decay and may increase the mineral density of certain bones, the routine fortification of water remains controversial because excessive fluoride intake can lead to mottling and crumbling of teeth and poor bone quality (high mineral density does not necessarily mean high bone strength). It's impossible to know how much fluoridated water is being consumed by one person, and therefore difficult to know whether they will be ingesting toxic quantities over time, although the World Health Organization report that the minimal quantities added to drinking water do not constitute a public health concern.[4]

Potassium

One of the most important minerals in the body, potassium ensures the proper functioning of nerves and muscles, helps the body to regulate fluid and, most importantly for bone, maintains pH levels. It is an alkaline compound that neutralizes acids in the body that deplete bone.

How it works

Bones act as a reservoir of alkaline compounds (primarily calcium) that can be supplied to the bloodstream when needed to balance acids and restore pH levels: when blood becomes too acidic, bone breakdown begins, releasing calcium. Potassium drawn from our diet helps to prevent this breakdown by keeping blood acidity from rising – therefore sparing the bones from having to release calcium. Potassium may also reduce the amount of calcium excreted in urine, again diminishing the need to draw on bone deposits.

Sources

Potassium is found in abundance in fruit and vegetables, especially bananas and of course potatoes, which are named with a nod to their potassium content.

Requirements

Relative to some minerals, we need quite a lot of potassium every day – 3,500 milligrams – more than ten times the amount of magnesium needed. Provided that plenty of fruit and vegetables are eaten, this shouldn't be difficult, but data from the Food and Agriculture Organization of the United Nations has shown that most European countries do not reach the recommended five portions (around 400 grams) of fruit and vegetables per day with some, including Norway, the Netherlands and Iceland, getting only around half this.[5] Potassium's link with calcium means that it may be especially important for the bone health of people who have a low-calcium diet, such as those avoiding dairy.

Iron

Iron is a mineral that is best known for its role in the formation of haemoglobin, the compound in red blood cells that carries oxygen around the body, but it also has many enzymic functions. These functions include helping to metabolize vitamin D and to form collagen, both of which are vital for bone health.

How it works

While iron is essential for body processes, having too much iron (as a result of taking too many supplements or a disorder that affects iron metabolism) is as detrimental as having too little (anaemia). Iron levels influence the formation of osteoclasts and osteoblasts and also affect their activity in remodelling bone. It is important to maintain a careful balance, as having either iron deficiency or iron overload can disrupt the process of bone metabolism and weaken bones.

Sources

Iron, in the form of haem iron, can be gained from eating red meat and in the form of non-haem iron from eating beans, pulses, leafy green vegetables, dried fruit, nuts and seeds, and fortified foods. Haem iron is absorbed directly into the bloodstream, but absorbing iron from plant-based sources requires a process involving vitamin C.

Iron uses the same absorption pathways as several other minerals and as a result can be inhibited by calcium, zinc and magnesium. This means that if you are taking calcium supplements to improve bone health, it is best to take them separately from foods that contain iron.

White flour is fortified with iron in more than 80 countries worldwide, making white bread a fairly important source of iron for many.[6] Although wholemeal flour naturally contains iron, the phytates in the germ of whole grains are another thing that can interfere with absorption. For this reason, white bread is a better source of iron than wholemeal and is, somewhat counter-intuitively, better if you are trying to improve iron status.

Requirements

Iron deficiency is one of the few common nutrient deficiencies in the Western world. It is especially prevalent among teenage girls and women, as they need almost twice as much iron as men in order to cover losses during menstruation. It is especially important for bone health in teenage girls that sufficient iron levels are maintained, as this is the time when peak bone mass is reached. From the age of 11, girls need 14.8 milligrams of iron per day – the same amount as adult women; men need 8.7 milligrams per day.

Vitamin K

Vitamin K is essential for the functioning of proteins that help blood to clot and others that play a role in bone metabolism and bone strength.

How it works

In bones, vitamin K affects bone remodelling by promoting the creation of bone-building osteoblasts and activating proteins, particularly osteocalcin, which are involved in bone mineralization. There is often a correlation between vitamin K deficiency and fractures and osteoporosis, indicating that it plays a significant role in bone strength.

Sources

In the diet sources include leafy green vegetables, broccoli, nuts and seeds, and oils and fats in smaller amounts.

Requirements

The recommendation for vitamin K intake is dependent on weight and is around 1 microgram per kilogram of body weight per day. However, because vitamin K is a fat-soluble vitamin, we don't actually need it every day, as we are able to store it in our bodies. It is thought that the average adult gets several hundred micrograms a day by eating a balanced diet and, as vitamin K is also produced in our bodies by several types of bacteria, deficiency is rare.

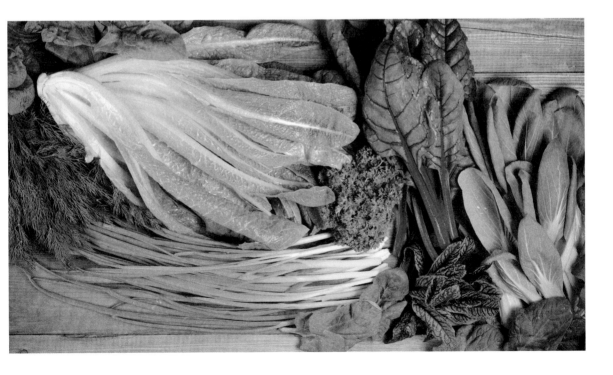

Boron

We have tiny amounts (3–20 milligrams) of the mineral boron in our bodies, but it is essential for the growth and maintenance of bones. Boron influences how bone uses calcium and magnesium, and also how hormones such as vitamin D and oestrogen work on bone cells. Boron appears to have an anti-inflammatory effect and may be helpful in reducing the symptoms of rheumatoid arthritis and osteoarthritis.

How it works

Although boron has been shown to confer benefits on bone health, the precise mechanisms by which it does this are still unclear. It appears to influence how the body processes other minerals – reducing the excretion of calcium and magnesium in the urine for example – which prevents bone demineralization. It also appears to increase oestrogen levels in older adults and extend the activity of vitamin D in the body.

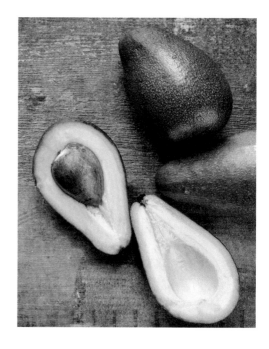

Sources

Plants provide the best sources of boron, in particular nuts, legumes, avocados and grapes, which contain 1–4.5 milligrams per 100 grams. Wine, cider, beer and water in some areas may also contain boron, and depending where the food is grown, fruit and vegetables too.

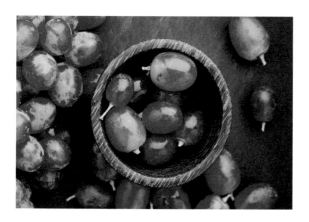

Requirements

There are no established recommended amounts for boron intake from food sources, although ingesting too much boron via supplements is harmful. It is thought that 1–3 milligrams per day, which is easily obtainable by following a varied diet, is sufficient for bone health.

Manganese

We need small amounts of the mineral manganese for the formation and maintenance of bone. Manganese plays an important role in the production of the collagen needed for bone formation and in the mineralization of bone. It also contributes to the structural components that form cartilage.

How it works

Working with copper, zinc, magnesium and calcium, manganese contributes to bone mineral density and ensures that bone remains strong. Manganese deficiency appears to be a risk factor for osteopoenia and osteoporosis.

Sources

Whole grains, legumes, leafy vegetables, dried fruit and nuts are all good sources of manganese, as is tea.

Requirements

There is no recommended dietary amount for manganese, but deficiency is rare, which indicates that most people get enough from their diet. In fact, deficiency is really only seen where manganese is deliberately restricted in the diet. Symptoms of deficiency include bone malformation and, among other things, changes in hair colour.

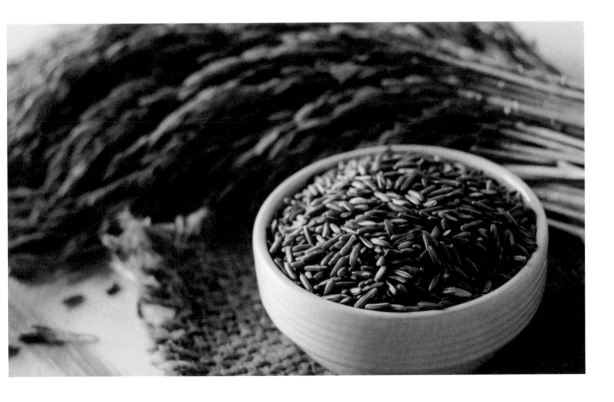

Phytonutrients

In addition to vitamins and minerals that are beneficial to health, plant-based foods such as fruit, vegetables, whole grains, tea and spices contain chemical compounds called phytonutrients which have antioxidant and anti-inflammatory properties and can neutralize harmful free radicals. This is one reason why eating fresh fruit and vegetables is better for your health than just taking supplements.

One group of phytonutrients called polyphenols has been shown to notably improve bone health through their antioxidant and anti-inflammatory actions and also because they increase the production of osteoblasts and reduce that of osteoclasts. Eating several

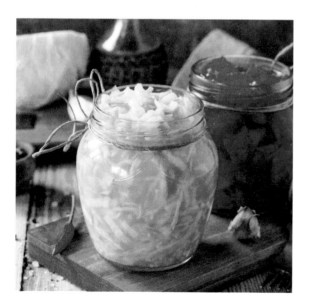

portions of fruit and vegetables every day has been shown to increase bone mineral density and reduce the risk of fractures. There has been extensive research into whether phyto-oestrogens (another type of phytonutrient found in foods such as soya), which mimic the action of oestrogen in the body, can protect bones, but numerous studies have found no link to improved bone health even with very high intakes of foods containing these compounds.

Probiotics and prebiotics

Good gut health is closely connected to bone health, as beneficial bacteria in our intestine perform a range of functions linked to the growth and maintenance of bone (see also pages 23–24). Beneficial bacteria can improve the absorption of vital bone-building nutrients and minerals such as calcium; regulate our immune response by excreting anti-inflammatory compounds; produce necessary substances such as vitamin K; and influence the action of hormones such as oestrogen and cortisol that affect bone health.

While there is a genetic component to our gut microbiome, we can take steps to alter the balance of the microorganisms that populate our gut by improving our diet to include foods that promote good bacteria. Consuming a wide range of fruit, vegetables, whole grains, beans and legumes is the best way to do this. These foods contain compounds known as prebiotics which stimulate the growth and activity of beneficial bacteria. You can also improve your microbiome by exercising, getting enough sleep, getting out into different natural environments, such as woods and farms, and by being around animals.

Another way to improve gut health is to take probiotics. These are live bacteria – lactobacilli and bifidobacteria – that are naturally created by the process of fermentation occurring in foods such as kefir, yogurt, kimchi and sauerkraut. There is some evidence to suggest that improving gut health by taking probiotics can help to slow the bone loss associated with osteoporosis.

Omega-3

Omega-3 acids are fats that we are unable to manufacture in our bodies, so must take in through our diet. These fats appear to increase the amount of calcium we absorb, inhibit bone breakdown, and have an anti-inflammatory effect. Their positive effect on inflammation has led to their use in conditions such as heart disease and rheumatoid arthritis, which also cause bone loss. Foods high in omega-3 fatty acids include oily fish such as salmon, mackerel and sardines, but they can also be found in nuts and seeds, especially walnuts and flaxseeds.

Are supplements helpful?

In general, it is always better to try and ensure you get adequate nutrients for bone health from dietary sources (see the requirements listed under individual vitamins and minerals) rather than from supplements, unless you have an underlying medical condition that necessitates their use. In some limited circumstances – such as people with limited sun exposure – vitamin D supplementation is recommended (*see page 62*), but other supplements may not provide any benefit.

Multivitamins, for example, contain a broad spectrum of micronutrients, but some nutrients interact with each other (calcium can block the absorption of magnesium, for example) so you may not gain any benefit to your bones. The benefit of fish oils is also unclear: while omega-3 fats found in fish oils have anti-inflammatory effects, there is currently little evidence that these supplements enhance bone health.

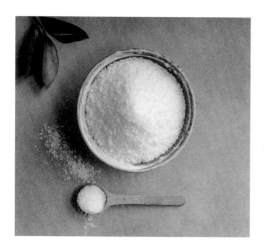

with higher fracture risk so adhering to the recommended level of less than 6 grams salt a day is still a good idea.

Sugar

Emerging evidence suggests that too much sugar may be bad for bones in several ways.[7] Sugar appears to lower calcium and magnesium absorption and deplete minerals from bone. It can also inhibit the activation of vitamin D and the action of bone-building osteoblasts, increasing the action of osteoclast action at the same time. This is related to increased inflammation and the production of excess insulin. The World Health Organization guidelines for sugar consumption are less than five per cent of total calorie intake or less than 30 grams per day.

Salt

For a long time, a high salt intake was thought to be associated with increased calcium loss from the bones, because sodium excreted in the urine takes calcium with it. But more recent analysis of the evidence has found that this doesn't necessarily mean lower bone mineral density because other mechanisms such as increased absorption of calcium from the diet can compensate for this extra excretion. A large study of post-menopausal women found no impact of a high-salt diet on fracture risk. A high-salt diet can, however, cause other problems such as high blood pressure, which can negatively affect calcium metabolism, and an increased risk of stroke and heart attacks – which are themselves associated

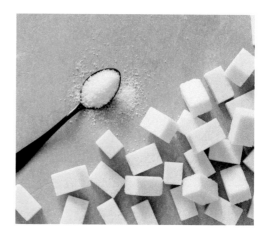

Alcohol

Alcohol interferes with vitamin D synthesis and a number of processes linked to calcium, which is a two-fold blow for bone health given that both compounds are necessary for bone growth (*see page 25*). Excess alcohol use can also affect balance, so is associated with an increased risk of falls and bone fractures. Sticking to under 14 units of alcohol per week is unlikely to affect your bones, but if you do drink more than this, it is advisable to cut down.

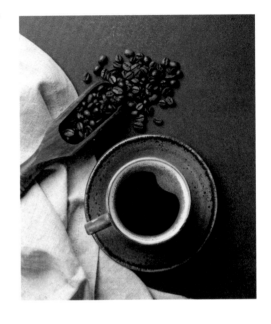

Saturated fat

Some dietary fats are needed because they help in the absorption or transportation of vitamins such as K and D in our bodies, which are necessary for bone health. However, consuming too much saturated fat can reduce the mineral density and mass of our bones. This type of fat can cause inflammation and affect calcium absorption and the production of bone-building osteoblasts. Saturated fat is generally solid at room temperature and includes coconut oil, butter, whole milk, cream, cheese and fat from cuts of meat; baked goods such as cakes and biscuits often contain high levels of saturated fat.

Caffeine

Guidelines on caffeine consumption in relation to bone health remain controversial because it can increase the excretion of calcium in urine. While tea, despite its caffeine content, is known to have a positive effect on bones because of its high phytonutrient content, it was thought that the high caffeine content in coffee might lead to the loss of bone density in older women. Recent studies, however, have indicated that drinking up to four cups of coffee per day is unlikely to affect bone mineral density.[8] If you do drink more than this and you have other risk factors for developing osteoporosis, increasing your calcium intake may be a good idea.

DIETS THAT IMPACT BONE HEALTH

There is no shortage of diets to follow, whether for weight loss, health or ethical reasons, but diets that are too restrictive or exclude whole food groups can be detrimental to bone health, particularly if undertaken during critical windows such as adolescence or the menopause. Below are some of the more common diets and how they may affect bone health.

The Mediterranean diet

Inflammation, and the steroids used to treat it, have such a detrimental effect on bone health that it's sensible to take steps to minimize inflammatory responses. The so-called Mediterranean diet is an anti-inflammatory diet that is generally accepted as being very good for overall health, as well as for our bones. It lowers the risk of developing non-communicable inflammatory diseases such as type 2 diabetes and heart disease, keeps bones strong and may even protect against dementia.

The diet consists of plenty of fresh fruit and vegetables, nuts and seeds, beans and legumes, whole grains, fish and low-fat dairy or dairy alternatives. Consuming a variety of these foods provides all the vitamins, minerals, fats and fibre needed for strong bones.

What you don't eat on this diet is almost as important as what you do eat. Most of your carbohydrate intake should come from whole grains such as wholemeal bread and pasta, brown rice and bulgur wheat, which have a high fibre content and anti-inflammatory properties. This means eating fewer refined carbohydrates like white rice, white bread, cakes and biscuits, which contain less fibre and can cause spikes in blood sugar, leading to fat storage around the abdomen, which in turn releases inflammatory compounds.

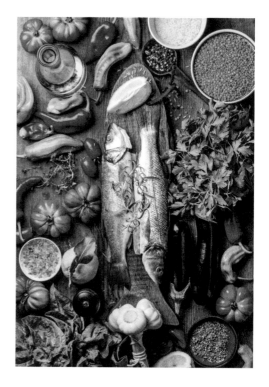

Protein in this diet is mostly sourced from beans, legumes and fish rather than meat, as lamb and fatty cuts of pork and beef can be high in saturated fat. Butter and saturated fats (including coconut oil) are also avoided in favour of unsaturated fats such as olive oil.

Vegetarian and vegan diets

A vegetarian diet that excludes meat and fish but includes eggs and dairy products can be similar to the Mediterranean diet – with the same benefits for bone health – but it is of course possible to eat an unhealthy vegetarian diet by still consuming lots of refined carbohydrates and very little in the way of vegetables.

The exclusion of dairy products and eggs from vegan diets mean that protein and calcium for bone health must be sourced elsewhere. The best sources include beans, lentils, tofu and fortified products such as milk alternatives and cereals. Both vegan and vegetarian diets should also include plenty of beans, lentils and whole grains to ensure that enough iron and zinc are consumed for bone health. This is particularly important for teenagers, who often experiment with vegetarian and vegan diets, as without adequate protein, calcium, iron and zinc they will not gain sufficient nutrients to achieve a good peak bone mass.

Although many vegan alternatives are now available, it is also worth noting that they may not provide the same nutrients as a non-vegan version. Depending on the recipe, vegan 'cheese' is a good example of this: if it is made from coconut oil, it may have similar textural properties to cheese, but will be low in both protein and calcium, so is not a direct substitution. Always check the nutritional panel and ingredients list to be clear about what's in these types of foods.

The alkaline diet

This diet has a controversial relationship with bone health. We know that the body closely controls acidity levels in the blood, maintaining its pH within strict margins. If blood becomes too acidic, calcium – which is alkaline – is released into the bloodstream to rebalance the pH (see also pages 59–60). This has obvious implications for bone health as bones are a reservoir for calcium; we also know that bone-breaking osteoclasts are activated by an acidic environment and bone-building osteoblasts prefer a more alkaline one. The premise of the alkaline diet is that if we eat fewer acid-forming foods, our bodies have to do less work to maintain bloodstream pH at the correct level, which includes our bones having to release less calcium.

However, the release of bone minerals is not the body's only method for neutralizing acid in the bloodstream:

the kidneys are the primary site for dealing with acidity as they filter out acids in the blood, excrete acids in the urine and produce bicarbonate (an alkaline compound), which acts as a buffer. We also remove acid in the form of carbon dioxide when we breathe out, so there are plenty of systems in place for managing this important task. Somewhat confusingly, acidic foods like lemon juice are not regarded as a problem in this diet, but rather foods that metabolize into acidic compounds such as meat, fish, eggs, dairy products, grains and alcohol. The alkaline diet proposes limiting these foods and eating mainly fruit, vegetables, carbohydrates (but not grains), fats and beans. This is not particularly unhealthy, but the exclusion of meat, fish and dairy products does limit vital sources of protein and calcium necessary for bone health, which may be a particular problem for older adults.

Controversy really centres on whether the alkaline diet has a proven positive effect on bone health. Some studies have implied that the diet has no beneficial effect on (and may even be detrimental to) bone density, while others have implied that eating an alkaline diet is useful for the treatment of osteoporosis.

It is possible that both arguments may be correct: kidney function declines with age, so it may be that as we age more of the burden of maintaining blood

pH falls to the bones so eating a more alkaline diet may mitigate this and therefore it becomes more important to consume a more alkaline diet. However, it is likely that other factors, such as body weight, adequate protein intake and physical activity, are still likely to be far more important in maintaining bone health than the alkaline content of our diet.

The Paleo diet

The Paleo diet is based on foods thought to have been eaten by our hunter-gatherer ancestors in the Paleolithic era. The premise is that our bodies have not yet evolved to cope with newer foods introduced by modern farming practices, and that we are therefore better suited to eating the same diet as early humans. This diet limits manufactured foods, including processed and farmed foods such as grains and beans, and also dairy products, which has implications for bone health.

While it is sensible to limit processed foods, the lack of grains and potatoes in this diet makes it very low in carbohydrates and means that the body has to derive most of its energy from fats and protein. Eating a large quantity of red meat to supply these needs can result in consuming high levels of saturated fat, which may increase inflammation in the body and can be detrimental to bone health.

In addition, removing grains and potatoes drastically reduces the amount of fibre consumed. Fibre is beneficial for gut bacteria and for reducing inflammation, both of which affect bone health (*see pages 23–24*). There is also evidence that grains were consumed long before they were farmed and that plenty of evolutionary changes have occurred to enable us to digest starches.

Avoiding dairy products means missing out on a source of calcium and removing beans and processed food as well gives little scope for consuming fortified products. Including tinned fish with bones, such as sardines, can go some way to boosting calcium levels, as can eating nuts, seeds and dark green leafy vegetables, but it can be difficult to ensure that intake is sufficient.

The ketogenic diet

This diet, similar to the Atkins and South Beach diets that preceded it, recommends limiting carbohydrate intake. These diets are generally followed in order to lose weight, but this can have a negative effect on bone density (*see pages 22–23*).

Weight loss occurs because restricting the amount of carbohydrates we eat forces our body to use stored fat (instead of carbohydrate) as an energy source. To do this, the body must produce compounds called ketones, which some organs can run on instead of using glucose.

The ketogenic diet is similar to the Paleo diet in that grains, potatoes and beans are only allowed in limited quantities because of their high carbohydrate content but, unlike the Paleo diet, dairy is permitted, so getting adequate calcium is less of an issue. There has been some suggestion, however, that ketosis (higher than normal blood acidity caused by the production of ketones) may encourage the bones to release alkaline minerals such as calcium in order to balance bloodstream pH levels. This would negatively impact bone density levels.

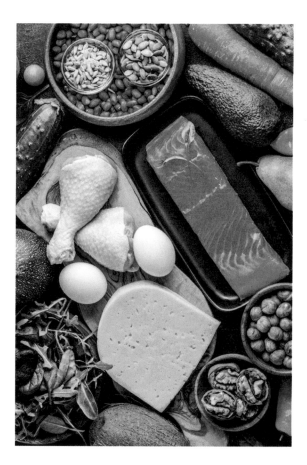

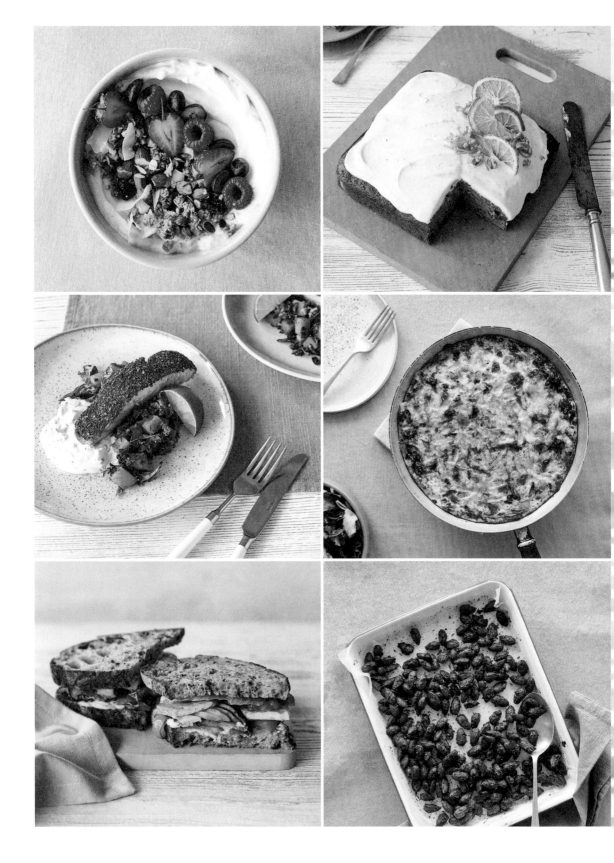

4

RECIPES

A healthy balanced diet, enriched with calcium and vitamin D, will help you build and maintain strong bones throughout your life. On the following pages you will find recipes that include the key ingredients and nutrients needed for bone health for all meals of the day – breakfast, lunch, main meals, sweets and snacks. They, along with the advice in the Nutrition section, will help you kickstart a dietary regime that supports your bones.

POWERSTART BREAKFAST SMOOTHIE

SERVES 4 | **PREP:** 10 minutes

A refreshing and surprisingly filling way to start the day, a smoothie is quick and easy when you are in a hurry and provides many of the valuable nutrients you need in a single glass. The yogurt, milk and almonds provide protein, but you can add 4 tablespoons of protein powder, if wished, as a boost.

2 ripe mangoes
300g (10oz) strawberries, hulled
2 bananas, peeled
125g (4½oz) 0% fat Greek yogurt
4 tbsp oat bran
1 tbsp ground flaxseeds
1tbsp chia seeds
30g (1oz) whole raw blanched almonds
1 tbsp clear honey or agave syrup
600ml (1 pint) chilled unsweetened soy
   milk, almond milk or semi-skimmed milk
ice cubes (optional)

1 Cut the mangoes in half and remove the peel and stone. Roughly chop the flesh and place in a blender with the strawberries, bananas, yogurt, oat bran, seeds, almonds, honey or agave syrup, and milk. If you want the smoothie to be really ice cold, add 4 ice cubes.

2 Blitz until everything is smooth and well combined. If the mixture is too thick for your liking, thin it with more milk or a little water.

3 Pour the smoothie into 4 glasses and drink immediately.

Tip: You can leave the smoothie in the blender jug and chill in the fridge for 1 hour. Don't leave it any longer or the banana will discolour.

Variations:

• Vary the fruit: try pineapple, kiwi fruit and apple for a green smoothie.
• Add kale or spinach.
• Peeled fresh root ginger will add heat, spice and a pungent, zingy taste.

SPINACH AND EGG TOASTIES

SERVES 4 | **PREP:** 5 minutes | **COOK:** 6–8 minutes

The eggs and bread provide protein while the spinach is a great way to get your daily iron and calcium. Tomatoes are a good source of vitamin C, as is the lemon juice, which will help your body to absorb the iron.

4 medium free-range eggs

olive oil, for brushing

1 garlic clove, crushed

400g (14oz) spinach leaves, trimmed
   and washed

a squeeze of lemon juice

4 sprigs cherry tomatoes on the vine

4 slices wholemeal, multigrain or
   multiseed bread

balsamic vinegar, for drizzling

salt and freshly ground black pepper

Tip: Crack each egg, one at a time, into a bowl or saucer before sliding into the pan, just in case one breaks when you crack it into the hot water. If you add a drop of white vinegar to the poaching water, the egg white will cook more quickly.

Variations:

- Substitute shredded kale for the spinach and cook for an extra
  2–3 minutes.
- Sprinkle with crushed chilli flakes or top with hollandaise sauce.
- Serve with grilled mushrooms.

1 Poach the eggs in an egg poacher if you have one. Alternatively, bring some water to the boil in a wide saucepan, reduce the heat to a bare simmer and gently crack the eggs into the hot water. Cover and leave to cook over the lowest possible heat for 3–4 minutes until the whites are set but the yolks are still runny. Carefully remove the eggs with a slotted spoon and drain on kitchen paper.

2 Meanwhile, lightly brush a saucepan with oil and cook the garlic over a low heat for 1 minute without browning. Add the spinach leaves, cover and cook for 1–2 minutes, shaking the pan occasionally until the spinach wilts and looks bright green. Stir in the lemon juice and season with salt and pepper.

3 Cook the tomatoes under a preheated overhead grill or in an oiled griddle pan until just softened and slightly charred.

4 Lightly toast the bread and place 1 slice on each plate. Cover with the spinach and drizzle with balsamic vinegar. Top with the eggs and serve immediately with the tomatoes.

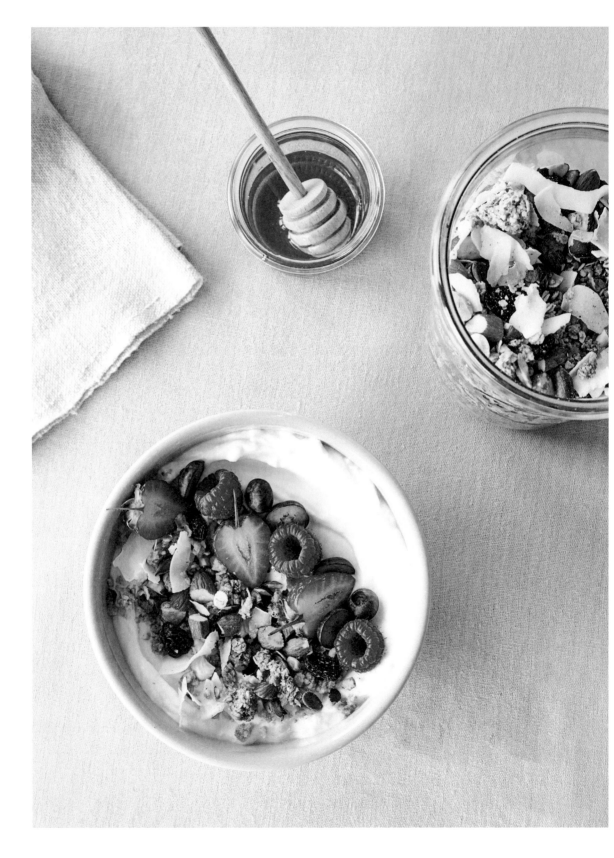

GRANOLA WITH SUMMER BERRIES

SERVES 4 | **PREP:** 10 minutes | **COOK:** 20–25 minutes

The granola in this recipe makes enough for approximately 12 servings, so store the rest in an airtight container for up to one month. Because it is relatively low in sugar and the carbs (oats) are low GI (glycaemic index), it gives you long-lasting energy without creating spikes in blood sugar levels.

500g (1lb 2oz) 0% fat Greek yogurt
350g (12oz) summer berries, such as strawberries, blueberries, raspberries
honey and coconut flakes, to serve

Granola:

4 tbsp sunflower oil
30g (1oz) coconut oil
4 tbsp clear honey
a few drops of vanilla extract
250g (9oz) rolled jumbo oats
60g (2oz) coarsely chopped almonds
60g (2oz) chopped hazelnuts
100g (3½oz) raisins
30g (1oz) pumpkin seeds
30g (1oz) sunflower seeds
½ tsp ground cinnamon

....

Tip: Vegans can substitute maple syrup for the honey and serve with dairy-free yogurt.

....

Variations:

• Add dried cherries, cranberries, sultanas or diced dried apricots.
• Serve with poached rhubarb, fresh sliced peaches or banana.

1 Preheat the oven to 170°C (150°C fan/325°F/Gas 3). Line a large baking tray with parchment paper.

2 Make the granola: heat the oils and honey in a pan set over a low heat, stirring gently to blend. Add the remaining ingredients, except for the raisins, and stir until well coated. Remove from the heat.

3 Spread the mixture evenly over the lined baking tray. Bake in the preheated oven for 20–25 minutes, stirring once or twice, until golden brown and crisp. Leave to cool, stir in the raisins, and store in an airtight container.

4 Divide the yogurt and berries between 4 serving bowls. Sprinkle 2–3 tablespoons granola over the top. Serve immediately topped with coconut flakes, if wished, and drizzled with honey.

ONE-PAN STOVETOP VEGGIE BRUNCH

SERVES 4 | **PREP:** 15 minutes | **COOK:** 20–25 minutes

This easy one-pan meal is a great way to start the day but can also be enjoyed for supper. Use the freshest, best-quality ingredients you can find and add any leftover vegetables or cheese lurking in the back of your fridge. It combines all the essential nutrients you need for good bone health.

2 tbsp olive oil

1 red onion, finely chopped

2 garlic cloves, crushed

1 fresh red chilli, finely chopped (optional)

250g (9oz) mushrooms, sliced

250g (9oz) halloumi, cubed

250g (9oz) cherry tomatoes, halved

450g (1lb) baby spinach leaves

4 medium free-range eggs

200g (7oz) Greek yogurt

1 tsp za'atar

sea salt and freshly ground black pepper

toasted pita or flatbreads, to serve

....

Tip: Vegans can substitute tofu for the halloumi and use dairy-free yogurt.

....

Variations:

- Sprinkle with paprika or drizzle with hot sauce, such as Sriracha.
- Add fresh chopped parsley, dill or coriander.
- Instead of halloumi, sprinkle the finished dish with grated Cheddar and flash it under a preheated hot grill.

1 Heat the olive oil in a large frying pan set over a medium heat. Cook the onion, garlic and chilli (if using), stirring occasionally, for 6–8 minutes or until they start to soften. Add the mushrooms and cook for 3–4 minutes until tender and golden.

2 Add the halloumi and cook, stirring and turning, for 3–4 minutes until golden brown and crusty.

3 Stir in the tomatoes and spinach and cook for 2–3 minutes more until the spinach wilts and the tomatoes are tender. Season to taste with salt and pepper.

4 Make 4 hollows in the mixture and crack an egg into each one. Reduce the heat to as low as it will go, then cover the pan and cook for 5 minutes, or until the egg whites are set but the yolks are still runny.

5 Drop spoonfuls of yogurt between the eggs and lightly dust with za'atar. Serve immediately with toasted pita or flatbreads on the side.

REFRIED BEAN BURRITOS

SERVES 4 | **PREP:** 10 minutes | **COOK:** 8 minutes

These tasty burritos work equally well as a simple light lunch or supper. So versatile, you can add everything from sliced avocado to cooked leftover vegetables, griddled chicken and tofu. The refried beans, cheese and tortillas provide protein as well as bone-healthy vitamins and minerals.

olive oil, for brushing

a bunch of spring onions, chopped

1 red chilli, finely chopped

1 x 400g (14oz) can refried beans

a handful of fresh coriander, chopped

4 large wholewheat tortillas

a large handful of crisp lettuce, such as cos or iceberg, shredded

4 heaped tbsp hot tomato salsa

100g (3½oz) Cheddar cheese, coarsely grated

salt and freshly ground black pepper

Greek yogurt or sour cream, to serve

....

Tip: The refried bean mixture should not be too thick as you need to spread it over the tortillas. Add more water if necessary to get the desired consistency.

....

Variations:

· Use as a filling for warm pita pockets or baked jacket potatoes.

· If you don't have refried beans, coarsely mash some drained canned kidney beans or black beans.

1 Lightly brush a non-stick frying pan with oil and set over a low to medium heat. Cook the spring onions and chilli, stirring occasionally, for 3 minutes or until softened. Stir in the refried beans and 2–3 tablespoons cold water. Heat through gently for about 5 minutes and then add the coriander and seasoning to taste.

2 Meanwhile, warm the tortillas in the oven or on a lightly oiled griddle pan set over a low heat.

3 Spread the refried bean mixture over the warm tortillas and cover with the lettuce, tomato salsa and Cheddar cheese.

4 Roll up the tortillas or fold the ends in to enclose the filling and then roll. Serve immediately with Greek yogurt or sour cream.

SMOKED SALMON AND GUACAMOLE SCRAMBLED EGG WRAPS

SERVES 4 | **PREP:** 15 minutes | **COOK:** 4–6 minutes

This easy weekend brunch provides protein, vitamins D and K and several essential minerals plus omega-3 fatty acids for promoting joint and heart health. The guacamole gives the wraps a spicy kick.

8 medium free-range eggs

60ml (2fl oz) milk

2 tsp butter

150g (5½oz) sliced smoked salmon, chopped

a small bunch of chives, snipped

4 wholewheat or multiseed wraps

salt and freshly ground black pepper

Greek yogurt and hot sauce, to serve (optional)

Guacamole:

½ red onion, diced

1 fresh green chilli, diced

1 garlic clove, crushed

½ tsp sea salt flakes

2 ripe avocados, peeled and stoned

juice of 1 lime

a small bunch of fresh coriander, chopped

Tip: If you don't have any wraps, serve the scrambled eggs on toast with the guacamole on the side.

Variation:
• Add chopped tomatoes and mushrooms.

1 Make the guacamole: crush the red onion, chilli, garlic and salt in a pestle and mortar. Mash the avocado flesh roughly with a fork – it shouldn't be too smooth. Stir in the lime juice, coriander and crushed onion mixture. Season with black pepper.

2 Beat the eggs and milk in a bowl until well blended. Season lightly with salt and pepper.

3 Place a non-stick saucepan over a low heat. Melt the butter and pour in the beaten egg mixture. Stir gently with a wooden spoon for 2–3 minutes and then fold in the smoked salmon and chives. Continue stirring for 1–2 minutes until the eggs scramble and set. Remove from the heat.

4 Meanwhile, heat the wraps in a low oven, a microwave or a griddle pan. Divide the scrambled eggs between them and add a large spoonful of guacamole. Fold over or roll up and eat immediately with yogurt and hot sauce, if using.

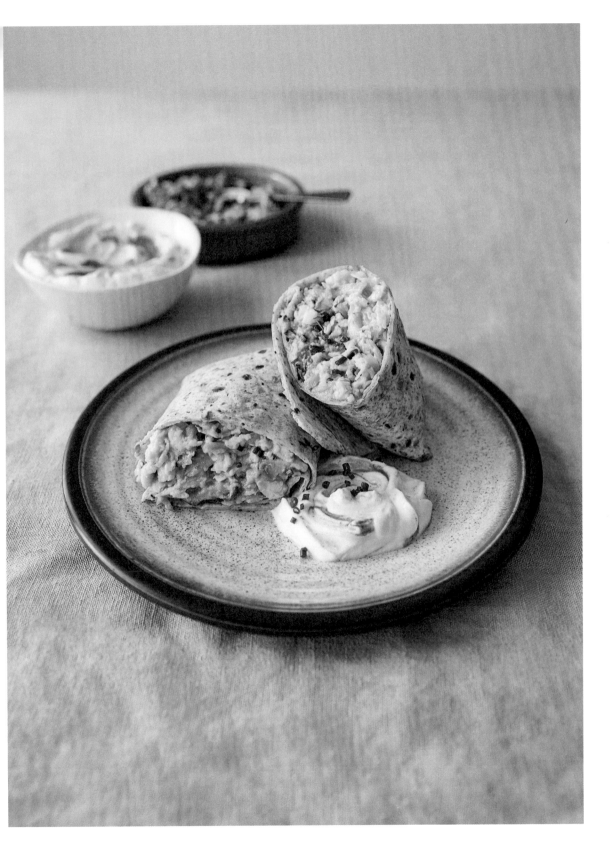

PUMPKIN AND BUTTER BEAN SOUP

SERVES 4 | **PREP:** 20 minutes | **COOK:** 40–45 minutes

Pumpkin is a great source of dietary fibre and vitamins A, B, C and E, while butter beans are among the richest sources of vegetarian protein and include magnesium, calcium, iron, copper and zinc for healing and repair.

2 tbsp coconut oil

1 onion, chopped

900g (2lb) pumpkin, peeled, deseeded and cubed

2 large carrots, finely chopped

2.5cm (1in) piece fresh root ginger, peeled and chopped

1 tsp ground cumin

1 tsp ground turmeric

2 tsp coriander seeds, toasted and crushed

1 litre (1¾ pints) hot vegetable stock

1 x 400g (14oz) can butter beans, rinsed and drained

salt and freshly ground black pepper

Spicy topping:

2 tbsp sunflower oil

1 small red onion, thinly sliced

2 garlic cloves, thinly sliced

1 red chilli, deseeded and shredded

1 tsp yellow mustard seeds

1 tsp cumin seeds

....

Variations:

• Substitute butternut squash or sweet potato for the pumpkin.

• Swirl a spoonful of Greek yogurt into each bowl.

1 Heat the coconut oil in a large pan and cook the onion over a low heat, stirring occasionally, for 6–8 minutes or until tender but not coloured. Add the pumpkin and carrots and cook gently, stirring occasionally, for 4–5 minutes until golden all over. Stir in the ginger, spices and seeds, and cook for 1 minute more.

2 Add the hot stock and bring to the boil. Reduce the heat, cover the pan and simmer gently for 20 minutes until the vegetables are tender. Add the beans and heat through gently.

3 Meanwhile, make the topping: heat the oil in a frying pan over a medium heat and cook the onion, stirring frequently, for 6–8 minutes, or until tender, crisp and golden brown. Turn up the heat and add the garlic, chilli and seeds. Cook for 1 minute or until the mustard seeds start popping. Remove from the heat.

4 Blitz the soup in a blender or food processor until smooth. Season to taste and reheat gently.

5 Ladle the hot soup into bowls and sprinkle the spicy topping over the top. Serve immediately.

HOMEMADE BEANS ON TOAST

SERVES 4 | **PREP:** 5 minutes | **COOK:** 10–15 minutes

This may seem a bit complicated but it's so much more tasty and healthier than the canned variety. Beans are an excellent source of plant protein and dietary fibre as well as bone-building calcium, iron and potassium.

2 tbsp olive oil

1 onion, finely chopped

2 garlic cloves, crushed (optional)

400g (14oz) cherry or baby plum tomatoes, diced

1 tbsp tomato paste

1 tsp sugar

1 x 400g (14oz) can butter beans, rinsed and drained

a few drops of balsamic vinegar

4 slices wholemeal or multigrain bread

salt and freshly ground black pepper

chopped fresh parsley or basil, to serve

1 Heat the oil in a saucepan set over a low to medium heat. Add the onion and garlic, if using, and cook for 6–8 minutes, stirring occasionally, until softened but not browned.

2 Add the tomatoes and cook for 3–4 minutes. Stir in the tomato paste, sugar and beans, and heat through gently. Add the balsamic vinegar and season to taste.

3 Lightly toast the bread and divide between 4 serving plates. Top with the beans, sprinkle with the chopped herbs and serve.

Tip: Don't worry if you don't have any fresh tomatoes; use the same weight of canned chopped tomatoes instead.

Variations:

- Try chickpeas, cannellini or red kidney beans.
- Spice it up with a diced chilli or some crushed chilli flakes.

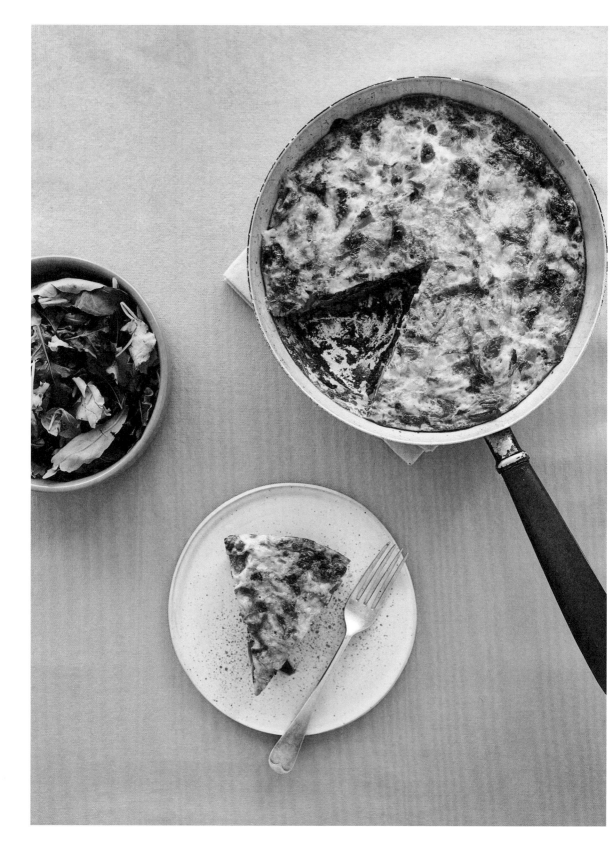

SQUASH AND SPINACH TORTILLA

SERVES 4 | **PREP:** 15 minutes | **COOK:** 25–30 minutes

This is a tortilla in the Spanish sense – a thick, creamy omelette filled with delicious vegetables and usually eaten lukewarm or at room temperature. Eggs are a good way of getting vitamin D as well as protein.

500g (1lb 2oz) butternut squash, peeled and cubed

3 tbsp olive oil

1 large red onion, chopped into wedges

2 red peppers, deseeded and cut into chunks

2 garlic cloves, crushed

1 red chilli, finely chopped (optional)

225g (8oz) spinach, washed and shredded

6 medium free-range eggs

60ml (2fl oz) milk

60g (2oz) grated cheese, such as Cheddar or Parmesan

salt and freshly ground black pepper

crisp green salad, to serve

....

Tip: Be sure to drain the squash well before adding it to the pan, so it does not release moisture and water into the egg mixture.

....

Variations:

- Use pumpkin or sweet potato instead of butternut squash.
- Substitute cooked kale or spring greens for the spinach.

1 Cook the butternut squash in a saucepan of boiling water for 5 minutes, or until it's just tender but still holds its shape. Drain well.

2 Heat the oil in a large non-stick frying pan over a low to medium heat and cook the onion, red pepper and garlic, stirring occasionally, for 6–8 minutes until softened but not browned. Add the chilli, if using, drained butternut squash and spinach and cook for 3–4 minutes, stirring occasionally, until the spinach wilts.

3 Beat the eggs and milk in a bowl and season lightly with salt and pepper. Pour into the frying pan and reduce the heat to a simmer. Cook gently for 5 minutes, until the tortilla is barely set in the middle and golden brown underneath.

4 Sprinkle with grated cheese and pop the pan under a preheated hot grill for about 5 minutes or until the top is lightly browned.

5 Slide the cooked tortilla out of the pan onto a wooden board and leave it to cool a little. Cut into wedges and serve with a crisp salad.

GREEK SPINACH HORTA SALAD

SERVES 4 | **PREP:** 20 minutes | **COOK:** 10 minutes

In Greece there is no set recipe for horta (boiled greens). People just gather seasonal green leaves, weeds and herbs, including spinach, young nettles, dandelion leaves and amaranth, and eat them warm or cold dressed with fruity olive oil and lemon. This recipe will boost your iron and vitamin K.

250g (9oz) cherry or baby plum
  tomatoes, halved
extra-virgin olive oil, for drizzling
175g (6oz) feta cheese, crumbled
a handful of dill, chopped
crushed chilli flakes, for sprinkling

Filo triangles:

3 sheets filo pastry
45g (1½oz) butter, melted
2 tbsp sesame seeds

Spinach horta:

1kg (2¼lb) spinach, washed and trimmed
2-3 tbsp olive oil
juice of 1 lemon
salt and freshly ground black pepper

....

Variations:

• Use a mixture of spinach and other greens.
• Use fried or grilled halloumi instead of feta.
• Serve with toasted pita or flatbreads.

1 Preheat the oven to 200°C (180°C fan/400°F/Gas 6). Line a baking tray with baking parchment.

2 Make the filo triangles: place 1 sheet of filo pastry on a clean work surface and lightly brush both sides with melted butter. Lay another sheet on top and brush with melted butter, then cover with the last sheet and brush with the remaining butter. Cut into squares and then cut each square in half into triangles.

3 Sprinkle with sesame seeds and place on the lined baking tray. Bake for 8–10 minutes until crisp and golden brown. Leave to cool.

4 Meanwhile, make the spinach horta: steam the spinach for 2–3 minutes until it wilts and is bright green. Drain well, squeezing out any excess water. Transfer to a bowl and stir in the olive oil and lemon juice. Season and leave to cool.

5 Divide the horta between 4 serving plates. Top with the tomatoes and drizzle with olive oil. Sprinkle the feta, dill and chilli flakes over the top and serve with the filo triangles.

SALADE NIÇOISE WRAPS

SERVES 4 | **PREP:** 15 minutes | **COOK:** 8 minutes

This delicious light meal is packed with protein – the eggs, tuna and wraps are all good sources and they supply other vital bone-friendly nutrients. If you prefer, simply serve this as a salad with some crusty bread or boiled new potatoes on the side.

150g (5½oz) fine green beans, trimmed

4 medium free-range eggs

2 x 140g (5oz) cans tuna in spring water, drained

4 tbsp light mayonnaise

4 spring onions, chopped

4 wholemeal or multigrain wraps

85g (3oz) mixed salad leaves

4 ripe tomatoes, quartered or sliced

30g (1oz) black olives, stoned

freshly ground black pepper

Tip: You can take a wrap to work as a packed lunch. Just make it the evening before, wrap in foil and pop it in the fridge overnight.

Variations:

- Substitute baby spinach or rocket for the lettuce.
- Make the tuna mayo more piquant by adding chopped capers or anchovies.
- Serve the salad in pita pockets or on toast.

1 Cook the green beans in a pan of boiling water for 4 minutes, or until just tender but still firm to the bite. Drain and rinse under cold running water. Pat dry with kitchen paper.

2 Meanwhile, boil the eggs for 8 minutes. Remove from the pan with a slotted spoon and transfer to a bowl of cold water. When they are cold, peel them and cut into quarters or slices.

3 Mash the tuna lightly with a fork and mix with the mayonnaise and spring onions. Season with pepper.

4 Spread the wraps out on a clean work surface and divide the salad leaves, tomatoes and olives between them. Add the green beans, eggs and tuna mayo, and fold or roll the wraps around the filling. Eat immediately or wrap in kitchen foil and chill in the fridge until required.

ROAST CHICKEN AND RICE LUNCHBOX SALAD

SERVES 4 | **PREP:** 15 minutes | **COOK:** 15–20 minutes | **STAND:** 10 minutes

This salad is a delicious way of using up leftovers – any cooked meat works well as do cooked or canned beans. You can portion up the salad into sealed containers to eat as a packed lunch or take on a picnic.

300g (10oz) brown rice (dry weight)

3 cooked beetroot, cut into chunks

2 juicy oranges, peeled and cut into segments

250g (9oz) cold roast chicken, cut into chunks or strips

a large handful of baby spinach leaves

a bunch of fresh mint or coriander, coarsely chopped

100g (3½oz) feta cheese, crumbled

60g (2oz) walnuts, roughly chopped

pomegranate molasses (optional), for drizzling

Dressing:

3 tbsp olive oil

1 tbsp nam pla (Thai fish sauce)

juice of 1 lime or small lemon

1 red chilli, finely chopped

....

Tip: Any grains work well, including quinoa, couscous and bulgur wheat. Cook them according to the packet instructions.

....

Variations:

- Use goat's or blue cheese instead of feta.
- Try any fruit, nuts or herbs you have to hand. A sprinkle of pomegranate seeds looks great and adds crunch.

1 Cook the rice according to the instructions on the packet. Remove from the heat and set aside, still covered, for 10 minutes before fluffing up with a fork. Set aside to cool.

2 Meanwhile, make the dressing: mix all the ingredients together.

3 Transfer the rice to a large bowl and fork through the beetroot, orange segments and chicken. Add the spinach and chopped herbs and toss lightly in the dressing.

4 Divide between 4 shallow bowls and sprinkle with the feta and walnuts, then drizzle with pomegranate molasses, if using.

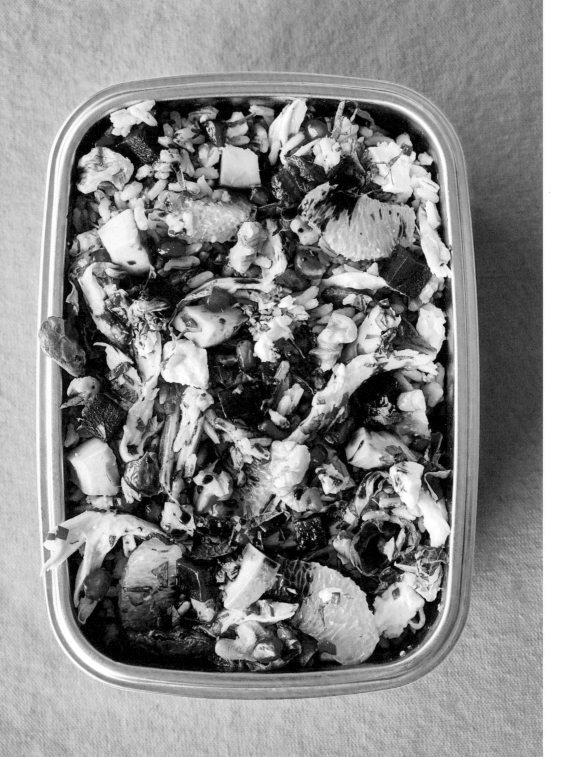

WARM LENTIL SALAD WITH PESTO

SERVES 4 | **PREP:** 15 minutes | **COOK:** 30 minutes

A lentil salad is a great way to get your daily protein and your five-a-day vegetables. Be sure to use Puy or green lentils rather than the smaller red ones, which collapse and go mushy when cooked.

225g (8oz) Puy or green lentils (dry weight)
1 vegetable stock cube or 1 heaped tsp bouillon powder
3 tbsp olive oil
1 large red onion, finely chopped
2 large carrots, finely chopped
3 sticks celery, finely chopped
3 garlic cloves, crushed
300g (10oz) cherry or baby plum tomatoes, halved
juice of 1 lemon
a handful of fresh flat-leaf parsley, chopped
2-3 tbsp balsamic vinegar
175g (6oz) fine green beans, trimmed and halved
140g (5oz) mozzarella, sliced
2 tbsp fresh green pesto
salt and freshly ground black pepper

Tip: This salad is best served warm or at room temperature.

Variations:
• Substitute goat's cheese or grilled halloumi for the mozzarella.
• Drizzle with hot sauce, balsamic glaze or harissa.

1 Put the lentils in a saucepan with enough cold water to cover them. Add the stock cube or bouillon powder and bring to the boil. Reduce the heat and simmer gently for 20 minutes, or until the lentils are just tender but still firm. Drain well, reserving the cooking stock.

2 Meanwhile, heat the oil in a large frying pan set over a low to medium heat. Cook the onion, carrots, celery and garlic, stirring occasionally, for 8–10 minutes, or until softened. Add the tomatoes and cooked lentils, and cook for 5 minutes, stirring occasionally. If the lentils start to stick or seem too dry, add a little of the reserved stock. Stir in the lemon juice, parsley and balsamic vinegar. Season to taste, and remove from the heat.

3 Cook the green beans in a pan of boiling water for 3–4 minutes, or until just tender. Drain and refresh under running cold water. Pat dry with kitchen paper.

4 Serve the lentil salad topped with the green beans and mozzarella, drizzled with pesto.

SWEET POTATO FISHCAKES

SERVES 4 | **PREP:** 15 minutes | **CHILL:** 30 minutes | **COOK:** 40–50 minutes

Sweet potatoes are a nutritional powerhouse, providing protein, carbs, vitamins B, C and E, as well as iron, zinc, potassium, magnesium, copper and phosphorus. Salmon provides protein, calcium, vitamin D and zinc.

800g (1¾lb) sweet potatoes, scrubbed

3 tbsp olive or sunflower oil, plus extra for frying

3 large leeks, washed, trimmed and thinly sliced

2 x 140g (5oz) cans salmon in spring water, drained and roughly flaked

a handful of fresh coriander, finely chopped

grated zest and juice of 1 lime

2 heaped tbsp plain flour, plus extra for dusting

salt and freshly ground black pepper

sweet chilli sauce, for drizzling

crisp green salad, to serve

....

Tip: You can make the fishcakes in advance and freeze for up to 3 months before defrosting them or cooking from frozen.

....

Variations:

· Use flaked cooked salmon or even smoked salmon trimmings.

· Vary the herbs: try parsley, dill or chives.

· Flavour with teriyaki or light soy sauce instead of lime juice.

1 Preheat the oven to 200°C (180°C fan/400°F/Gas 6).

2 Pierce the sweet potatoes with a fork. Place on a baking tray and bake for 30–40 minutes, or until tender. Remove and cool.

3 Meanwhile, heat the oil in a frying pan over a low heat and cook the leeks, stirring occasionally, for 6–8 minutes until soft but not coloured.

4 When the sweet potatoes are cool enough to handle, scoop out the insides and mix with the leeks, salmon, coriander and lime zest and juice. Stir in the flour to bind everything together and season with salt and pepper. If the mixture is not very firm, add more flour.

5 Divide into 8 portions and shape each one into a patty. Dust lightly with flour, then cover and chill in the fridge for 30 minutes.

6 Pour in enough oil to just cover the base of a large frying pan and set over a medium heat. Cook the fishcakes for 4–5 minutes on each side until golden brown and crispy. Remove and serve, drizzled with chilli sauce, with salad.

VEGAN QUINOA AND BEAN BURRITOS

SERVES 4 | **PREP:** 15 minutes | **COOK:** 20 minutes

These spicy vegan burritos are relatively low in carbs but full of healthy plant protein, dietary fibre, vitamins and minerals. If you're not a vegan, you can use grated Cheddar or Monterey Jack cheese and Greek yogurt.

300ml (½ pint) vegetable stock

100g (3½oz) quinoa (dry weight)

3 tbsp olive oil

1 large red onion, finely chopped

3 garlic cloves, crushed

2 red peppers, deseeded and chopped

1 fresh red chilli, diced

1 tsp ground cumin

1 x 400g (14oz) can black beans, rinsed
     and drained

200g (7oz) canned sweetcorn kernels in
     water, drained

juice of 1 lime

a handful of coriander, chopped

8 cornmeal tortillas

115g (4oz) grated dairy-free vegan cheese

salt and freshly ground black pepper

dairy-free coconut or soy yogurt and salsa or
     pico de gallo, to serve

....

Tip: You can buy dairy-free vegan cheese in most health food stores and supermarkets.

....

Variations:

• Add some thinly sliced or diced avocado to the burritos.

• Use red kidney beans instead of black.

1 Heat the stock in a saucepan and when it starts to boil, tip in the quinoa. Reduce the heat, cover and simmer gently for 15 minutes or until the quinoa is tender and most of the liquid has been absorbed. Turn off the heat and leave for 6–8 minutes to steam. Drain any excess liquid and fluff with a fork.

2 Meanwhile, make the filling: heat the oil in a frying pan set over a medium heat. Cook the onion, garlic, red peppers and chilli for 5 minutes. Add the cumin and cook for 5 minutes, stirring occasionally, until the vegetables have softened. Stir in the beans and sweetcorn and heat through gently. Stir in the quinoa, lime juice and coriander, and season to taste.

3 Preheat the grill to hot. Divide the filling between the tortillas and fold or roll them. Place them, seam-side down, in a foil-lined grill pan and sprinkle over the grated cheese.

4 Cook under the grill for 5 minutes or until the cheese melts and the tortillas are golden brown. Serve topped with yogurt and salsa.

CRUNCHY TOFU PAD THAI

SERVES 4 | **PREP:** 15 minutes | **COOK:** 10 minutes

Tofu is an excellent source of plant protein as it contains all eight essential amino acids. It is enlivened here with the hot, salty and zingy flavours of chilli, tamarind and lime juice. Firm or extra-firm tofu is easier to stir-fry.

250g (9oz) flat rice noodles (dry weight)
2 tbsp groundnut oil
3 garlic cloves, crushed
2.5cm (1in) piece fresh root ginger, peeled and diced
a bunch of spring onions, sliced
1 red bird's eye chilli, thinly sliced
175g (6oz) thin green beans, trimmed and halved
400g (14oz) extra-firm or firm tofu, cubed
100g (3½oz) bean sprouts
4 tbsp crushed roasted peanuts
2 tbsp sesame seeds
a handful of fresh coriander, chopped
lime wedges and sweet chilli sauce, to serve

Peanut butter sauce:
5 tbsp unsweetened crunchy peanut butter
3 tbsp soy sauce
1 tbsp nam pla (Thai fish sauce)
2 tbsp palm sugar
2 tbsp tamarind paste
grated zest and juice of 2 limes
2-3 tbsp water

1 Put all the ingredients for the peanut butter sauce in a bowl and mix until well blended.
2 Prepare the rice noodles according to the instructions on the packet.
3 Heat the oil in a wok or deep frying pan set over a medium to high heat. Add the garlic, ginger, spring onions and chilli and stir-fry briskly for 1 minute. Add the green beans and tofu and stir-fry for 4–5 minutes until the tofu is golden.
4 Stir in the peanut butter sauce, then reduce the heat, cover the pan and cook for 2 minutes. Add the rice noodles and bean sprouts and stir-fry for 1 minute, tossing them lightly in the sauce.
5 Divide the mixture between 4 shallow serving bowls. Sprinkle with the roasted peanuts, sesame seeds and coriander and serve with lime wedges for squeezing and some sweet chilli sauce.

Variation:
• Substitute broccoli or cauliflower florets for the green beans.

SEEDED ROASTED SALMON

SERVES 4 | **PREP:** 15 minutes | **COOK:** 25 minutes

Seeds are an important source of dietary fibre as well as vitamins A, B, C, E and K, calcium, copper, iron, magnesium, zinc and potassium (depending on the type). Kale contains iron, calcium, magnesium and vitamin K.

sunflower oil, for oiling

2 tsp black mustard seeds

1 tsp coriander seeds

2 tsp fennel seeds

1 tsp ground turmeric

4 x 140g (5oz) salmon fillets, skinned

4 tbsp 0% fat Greek yogurt

salt and freshly ground black pepper

Spicy sweet potatoes:

2 tbsp sunflower oil

1cm (½in) piece fresh root ginger, peeled and diced

1 red chilli, deseeded and shredded

1 tsp black mustard seeds

1 tsp cumin seeds

1 tsp ground turmeric

600g (1lb 5oz) sweet potatoes, peeled and cubed

4 medium tomatoes, coarsely chopped

400g (14oz) kale, washed, trimmed and shredded

juice of ½ lime

salt and freshly ground black pepper

....

Tip: You can also make this with skinned cod, haddock or sea bass fillets.

1 Preheat the oven to 180°C (160°C fan/350°F/Gas 4). Lightly oil a baking tray.

2 Set a frying pan over a medium heat and dry-fry the black mustard and coriander seeds for 1 minute until the mustard seeds begin to pop. Stir in the fennel seeds and cook for 30 seconds. Remove and grind the seeds coarsely in a pestle and mortar or electric grinder. Add the turmeric and salt and pepper.

3 Coat the salmon fillets with the ground toasted seeds, pressing them in gently. Place on the baking tray and cook in the preheated oven for 15–20 minutes, turning halfway through, until the crust is golden and the fish is cooked through.

4 While the fish is cooking, make the sweet potatoes. Heat the oil in a large frying pan set over a medium heat and cook the ginger, chilli and seeds for 2 minutes. Add the turmeric and sweet potatoes and cook for 5 minutes, stirring occasionally. Add 6 tablespoons water and the tomatoes, then cover and simmer gently for 10 minutes,

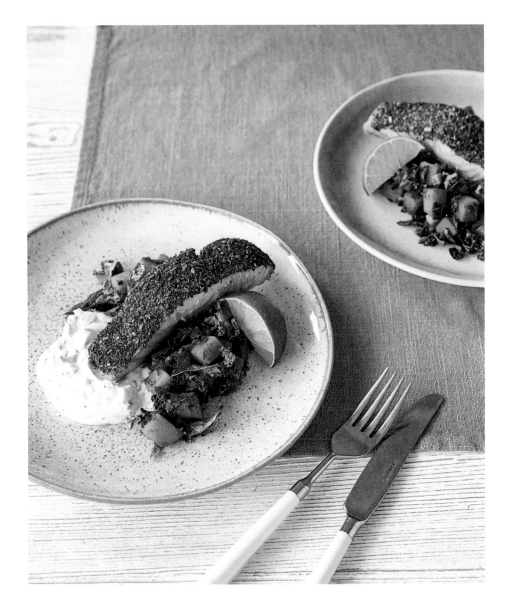

or until the potatoes are just tender. Stir in the kale and cook for 4–5 minutes until tender. Add the lime juice and season to taste.

5 Divide between 4 serving plates and top with a spoonful of yogurt. Serve immediately with the salmon fillets.

Variations:

- Use pumpkin or butternut squash instead of sweet potato.
- Substitute spinach or spring greens for the kale.

SPICED MACKEREL WITH GREEN RICE

SERVES 4 | **PREP:** 15 minutes | **CHILL:** 30 minutes | **COOK:** 25–30 minutes

An often under-rated and overlooked oily fish, mackerel is really delicious and healthy – full of protein and healthy omega-3 fats, which help to protect your heart. Here it is marinated in spicy yogurt before being grilled.

4 tbsp 0% fat Greek yogurt
1 tbsp curry paste
juice of ½ lime
4 mackerel fillets
500g (1lb 2oz) carrots, sliced
1 tsp ground cumin
1 tsp ground turmeric
a handful of fresh coriander, chopped
vegetable oil, for brushing
salt and freshly ground black pepper

Green rice:
225g (8oz) basmati rice (dry weight)
2 tbsp sunflower or rapeseed oil
3 garlic cloves, crushed
2.5cm (1in) piece fresh root ginger, peeled and grated
400g (14oz) shredded spring greens, green cabbage, kale or spinach
juice of 1 lime

Tip: You could cook salmon or white fish fillets in the same way.

Variations:
- Add black mustard seeds or a diced chilli to the stir-fried green rice.
- Substitute sweet potato for the carrots.

1 Mix the yogurt, curry paste and lime juice in a bowl. Slash the skin of the mackerel fillets 2–3 times with a sharp knife, and brush the yogurt mixture all over. Cover and chill in the fridge for 30 minutes
2 Cook the rice according to the instructions on the packet.
3 Meanwhile, cook the carrots in a pan of lightly salted boiling water for 12–15 minutes until tender. Drain well, mash with a fork and stir in the ground spices and coriander. Season to taste and keep warm.
4 Make the green rice: heat the oil in a wok or large frying pan over a medium to high heat. Stir-fry the garlic, ginger and greens for 2–3 minutes and then stir in the rice. Stir-fry for 2–3 minutes more, then stir in the lime juice. Keep warm.
5 Remove the mackerel from the marinade and cook in a foil-lined pan under a preheated hot grill for 2–3 minutes each side until cooked and the skin is crisp and golden, brushing with the leftover mixture. Serve immediately with the mashed carrots and green rice.

LEBANESE LEMON CHICKEN

SERVES 4 | **PREP:** 15 minutes | **COOK:** 50 minutes

The potatoes absorb most of the pan juices, lemon, garlic and olive oil, and taste amazing. Chicken thighs have more flavour than breasts and are not only packed with protein but also with the essential minerals iron, potassium and magnesium as well as vitamin B6.

675g (1½lb) new potatoes, such as Charlotte, halved or quartered
1 large onion, cut into wedges
8 chicken thighs
juice of 3 large lemons
5-6 tbsp olive oil
8 garlic cloves
1 lemon, sliced or cut into wedges
a good pinch of paprika
a handful of fresh flat-leaf parsley, chopped
salt and freshly ground black pepper
salad or cooked green vegetables, to serve

Tip: Serve accompanied by a small dish of fiery harissa for people to help themselves.

Variations:
- Add cherry or baby plum tomatoes after removing the foil.
- Use chicken legs or breasts instead of thighs.

1 Preheat the oven to 200°C (180°C fan/400°F/Gas 6).
2 Put the potatoes, onion wedges and chicken in a large shallow roasting pan. Mix together the lemon juice and olive oil. Peel and crush 3 garlic cloves and add to the mixture.
3 Pour over the chicken and vegetables in the pan, and tuck the unpeeled garlic cloves and lemon slices or wedges in between. Season with salt and pepper and dust with paprika, then cover the dish with kitchen foil.
4 Bake in the preheated oven for 30 minutes, then remove the foil and cook for 20 minutes, or until the potatoes are tender and browning, the onions are starting to caramelize, and the chicken is cooked through and the skin is golden brown and crispy. Slip the garlic out of the skins and sprinkle over the top with the parsley.
5 Divide between 4 serving plates and serve immediately with a crisp salad or some green vegetables.

BEEF KOFTAS WITH INDIAN SALAD

SERVES 4 | **PREP:** 15 minutes | **COOK:** 15 minutes

Cook the koftas on a barbecue over hot coals for a really smoky flavour, or under an overhead grill. For the best results, use really lean mince, which is a good source of bone-friendly protein, vitamin D, iron, zinc, magnesium, potassium and phosphorus. The crunchy Indian salad (kachumber) is delicately spiced and refreshing.

500g (1lb 2oz) minced beef (max. 5% fat)
1 red onion, grated
3 garlic cloves, crushed
1 fresh green chilli, diced
1 tsp ground cumin
1 tsp ground coriander
a handful of fresh coriander, chopped
olive oil, for brushing
250g (9oz) brown rice (dry weight)
salt and freshly ground black pepper

Indian salad:

½ cucumber, diced
1 small red onion, finely chopped
1 red pepper, deseeded and chopped
3 juicy tomatoes, chopped
1 fresh red or green chilli, deseeded and diced
a pinch of ground cumin
a handful of fresh coriander, chopped
a handful of fresh mint, chopped
juice of 1 lime or ½ lemon
sea salt flakes

1 Make the Indian salad: mix all the ingredients together in a bowl, adding sea salt to taste.

2 Put the minced beef, onion, garlic, chilli, ground spices and fresh coriander in a bowl with some salt and pepper. Mix together well and then, using your hands, mould the mixture into 12 sausage shapes around some skewers and brush lightly with oil.

3 Cook the koftas on a hot barbecue, turning them occasionally, for 7–10 minutes until evenly browned and slightly charred. Alternatively, lay them in a foil-lined grill pan and cook under a hot grill.

4 Meanwhile, cook the rice according to the instructions on the packet.

5 Serve the hot koftas immediately with the Indian salad and rice.

Tip: You can use wooden or metal skewers. If using wooden ones, soak them in water first to prevent them from burning.

Variations:
• Use minced lean lamb instead of beef.
• Serve with a spicy tomato or mango salsa.

DHAL WITH GRIDDLED VEGETABLES

SERVES 4 | **PREP:** 15 minutes | **COOK:** 35 minutes

This is real comfort food and combines lentils, which are a good source of vegetarian slow-release protein and carbohydrate, with sweet potatoes, which have a lower GI (glycaemic index) than white ones.

1 tbsp vegetable oil

3 garlic cloves, crushed

1 tsp peeled and grated fresh root ginger

1 red chilli, finely chopped

1 tsp black mustard seeds

1 tsp cumin seeds

1 tsp ground turmeric

1 tsp garam masala

250g (9oz) split red lentils (dry weight)

500ml (16fl oz) vegetable stock

1 x 400ml (14fl oz) can coconut milk

4 ripe tomatoes, chopped

100g (3½oz) baby spinach leaves

juice of 1 lime

naan bread, to serve

Spiced griddled vegetables:

1 large sweet potato, cut into thin wedges
  (skin left on)

2 red or yellow peppers, cut into chunks

2 tbsp sunflower or groundnut oil

1 tsp cumin seeds

1 red chilli, deseeded and cut into thin slices

8 fresh curry leaves

salt and freshly ground pepper

....

Tip: Don't use green or brown lentils - they will not break down into a thick paste.

1 Heat the oil in a saucepan and cook the garlic, ginger and chilli over a low to medium heat for 2 minutes. Stir in the seeds and ground spices, and when the mustard seeds start to pop, add the lentils, vegetable stock and coconut milk.

2 Bring to the boil, then reduce heat and simmer gently for 15 minutes. Add the tomatoes and simmer for 15 minutes more or until the dhal is thick and creamy. If it's still a bit liquid, cook for a little longer; if it's too thick, add some more stock.

3 When the dhal is nearly ready, put the sweet potato, peppers, oil and salt and pepper in a bowl and toss to coat. Heat a griddle pan until hot and cook the vegetables for 2–3 minutes each side, until tender and charred. Remove and keep warm.

4 Add the cumin seeds, chilli and curry leaves to the oil left in the pan and cook for 2 minutes. Spoon over the griddled vegetables.

5 Stir the spinach and lime juice into the dhal and season to taste. Divide between 4 shallow bowls, top with the vegetables and serve with naan.

SEEDY NUT BUTTER FLAPJACKS

MAKES 16 | **SOAK:** 10–15 minutes | **PREP:** 15 minutes | **COOK:** 20–25 minutes

Almond butter, substituted for melted dairy butter, works with the soaked dates, maple syrup and egg whites to bind the mixture. The healthiest of all the nut butters, it is a good source of protein and bone-friendly essential minerals, and has more dietary fibre and vitamin E and fewer calories.

100g (3½oz) stoned dates

¾ tsp bicarbonate of soda

150g (5½oz) smooth almond butter

2 egg whites

120ml (4fl oz) maple syrup

400g (14oz) jumbo porridge oats

1 tsp ground cinnamon

60g (2oz) chopped almonds

30g (1oz) sunflower seeds

30g (1oz) pumpkin seeds

a few drops of vanilla extract

Tip: You can buy almond butter in most supermarkets and health-food stores but it's easy to make at home. Just grind the almonds in a food processor into a thick, oily paste.

Variations:

• Use clear honey instead of maple syrup.

• Make the flapjacks with peanut, hazelnut or cashew butter.

• Add raisins or different nuts and seeds.

1 Preheat the oven to 180°C (160°C fan/350°F/Gas 4). Line a 30 x 20cm (12 x 8in) baking tin with baking parchment.

2 Put the dates and bicarbonate of soda in a bowl and pour some boiling water over the top. Stir and leave to soak for 10–15 minutes. Drain the dates, reserving the soaking liquid.

3 Place in a food processor with the almond butter, egg whites and maple syrup and blitz until smooth.

4 Transfer to a mixing bowl and stir in the porridge oats, cinnamon, almonds, seeds and vanilla. The mixture should be quite sticky; if it's too dry, stir in some of the reserved soaking liquid to get the desired consistency.

5 Spoon the mixture into the prepared tin and press it down with the back of a spoon to level the top. Bake in the preheated oven for 20–25 minutes until golden brown.

6 Remove from the oven and leave to cool in the tin before cutting into squares. Store in an airtight container for up to 5 days.

AUTUMN FRUIT CRUMBLE

SERVES 4 | **PREP:** 15 minutes | **COOK:** 30–40 minutes

Everybody loves crumble, especially in cooler months when autumn fruit is in season. The crunchy, nutty topping is made with nutritious oats and nuts to boost your daily protein, iron, zinc and magnesium.

butter, for greasing

675g (1½lb) plums or greengages

juice of 1 orange

2 tbsp water

3 tbsp caster sugar

a pinch of ground cinnamon

2 tbsp flaked almonds

pouring cream, crème fraîche, ice cream, custard or Greek yogurt, to serve

Crumble topping:

100g (3½oz) plain flour

85g (3oz) butter, diced

85g (3oz) Demerara sugar

60g (2oz) porridge oats

60g (2oz) ground almonds

....

Tip: You can use frozen and defrosted or bottled fruit instead of fresh.

....

Variations:

- Use peaches, nectarines or apricots instead of plums.
- Stew some damsons and add to the plums.
- Dot the plums with butter before covering with the crumble.

1 Preheat the oven to 180°C (160°C fan/350°F/Gas 4). Lightly butter a baking dish.

2 Make the crumble topping: put the flour in a large mixing bowl and rub in the butter with your fingertips until the mixture resembles fine breadcrumbs. Stir in the sugar, porridge oats and ground almonds. Add a few drops of water and stir in gently until the mixture starts to clings together.

3 Cut the plums or greengages in half and remove the stones. Put the fruit in the buttered baking dish and sprinkle over the orange juice, water, sugar and cinnamon.

4 Cover the fruit with the crumble topping right up to the edges of the dish. Scatter with the flaked almonds and bake in the preheated oven for 30–40 minutes, or until the topping is crisp and golden.

5 Serve hot with cold pouring cream, crème fraîche, ice cream, custard or thick Greek yogurt.

SPICED CARROT CAKE WITH ORANGE FROSTING

SERVES 8–10 | **PREP:** 20 minutes | **COOK:** 45–55 minutes

This is the easiest carrot cake you'll ever make; it's moist and delicious and high in protein with the eggs, yogurt and wholemeal flour. Vegetable oil is used instead of butter to reduce the saturated fat and make it healthier.

175g (6oz) raw cane or demerara sugar

175ml (6fl oz) sunflower oil, plus extra for greasing

3 medium free-range eggs, beaten

250g (9oz) carrots, grated

finely grated zest and juice of 1 orange

175g (6oz) wholemeal self-raising flour

1 tsp baking powder

1 tsp ground cinnamon

½ tsp grated nutmeg

60g (2oz) chopped walnuts

walnut halves or shredded orange zest, to decorate

Orange frosting:

115g (4oz) thick 0% fat Greek yogurt

115g (4oz) light soft cheese

2–3 tbsp icing sugar

grated zest of 1 orange

Tip: Instead of frosting the cake, dust with icing sugar. It will stay fresh in an airtight container in a cool place for up to 5 days.

Variation:

• Add sultanas to the cake mixture.

1 Preheat the oven to 180°C (160°C fan/350°F/Gas 4. Lightly oil a 20 x 20cm (8 x 8in) cake tin and line with baking parchment.

2 In a mixing bowl or food mixer, beat the sugar, oil and eggs until well blended. Mix in the grated carrots and orange zest. Sift in the flour and baking powder and mix well. Stir in the spices with most of the orange juice. Lightly stir in the walnuts, distributing them evenly throughout the mixture. Transfer to the lined cake tin and level the top.

3 Bake in the preheated oven for 45–55 minutes until the cake is well risen and a skewer inserted into the centre comes out clean. Cool in the tin and then turn out onto a wire rack.

4 Make the orange frosting: put all the ingredients, together with the leftover orange juice from the cake, into a bowl and mix until smooth and creamy. Spread the frosting over the top of the cake and decorate with some walnuts or orange zest.

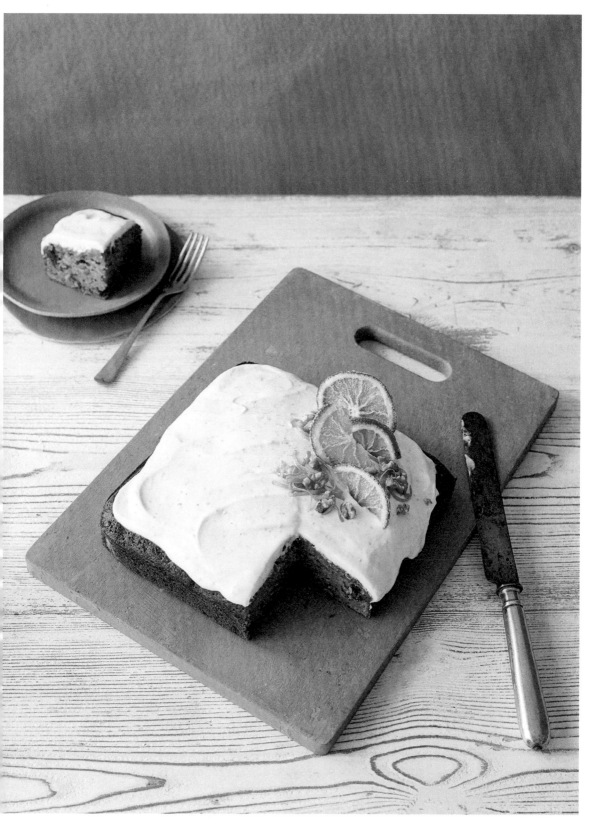

HOMEMADE HUMMUS

SERVES 4 | **PREP:** 15 minutes

A good source of vegetable protein and low in fat and cholesterol, chickpeas pack an impressive punch of minerals (iron, calcium, potassium, magnesium, manganese, zinc and selenium) plus vitamins B6, C and K to help build strong bones and promote a healthy gut and digestive tract.

2 x 400g (14oz) cans chickpeas

2-3 garlic cloves, crushed

4 tbsp tahini

1 tbsp extra virgin olive oil, plus extra
   for drizzling

juice and grated zest of 1 lemon, plus extra
   for drizzling

salt and freshly ground black pepper

finely chopped parsley for sprinkling

za'atar, paprika or sumac, for dusting
   (optional)

....

Tip: Serve this as a dip with toasted triangles of pita bread or raw vegetable crudités, as a spread for sandwiches or a filling for wraps.

....

Variations:

• Sprinkle with dukkah, crushed cumin or coriander seeds, crushed chilli flakes, toasted pine nuts, finely chopped red onion, or cooked caramelized onions.

• Stir in some 0% fat Greek yogurt to make the hummus more creamy.

• To flavour the hummus, blitz with roasted red peppers or root vegetables, fresh coriander or basil, or avocado and chilli.

1 Drain the chickpeas, reserving the liquid, and then rinse under running cold water. Pat them dry with kitchen paper.

2 Blitz in a blender or food processor with the garlic, tahini, olive oil and lemon juice to a rough purée.

3 Add some of the reserved chickpea liquid until you end up with the consistency you want. It should be quite soft (but not runny) and a little grainy, not too smooth. Season to taste with salt and pepper.

4 Transfer the hummus to a serving bowl and drizzle with olive oil and lemon juice. Sprinkle with parsley and dust, if wished, with za'atar, paprika or sumac.

CHICKEN CAESAR SANDWICH

SERVES 4 | **PREP:** 15 minutes

This sandwich makes a quick snack to enjoy at home or prepare it in advance and take it to work as a packed lunch. It's nutritious as well as delicious, providing you with bone-strengthening protein, vitamin D, calcium, zinc and phosphorus.

1 small cos lettuce, trimmed and leaves
   coarsely chopped
300g (10oz) cooked chicken breast,
   skinned and chopped
8 slices wholegrain or multiseed bread
60g (2oz) coarsely grated Parmesan cheese
freshly ground black pepper

Caesar dressing:
8 tbsp light mayonnaise
juice of ½ lemon
a dash of Worcestershire sauce
2-3 garlic cloves, crushed
8 anchovies, rinsed and chopped

1 Make the Caesar dressing: whisk all the ingredients together in a bowl until smooth.
2 Add the chicken and stir until everything is lightly coated. Add the lettuce and toss gently.
3 Divide the chicken and lettuce mixture between 4 bread slices. Sprinkle with the Parmesan and lightly season with black pepper. Drizzle any remaining dressing over the top. Cover with the remaining bread slices and cut in half or into quarters.

....

Tip: You can use wholemeal, multiseed or wholegrain rolls instead of bread, or use the chicken and lettuce as a filling for wraps or pita bread pockets.

....

Variations:
- Lightly toast the bread before adding the chicken and lettuce.
- Add some sliced tomatoes, roasted red pepper or mashed avocado.
- Substitute cooked turkey or prawns for the chicken.

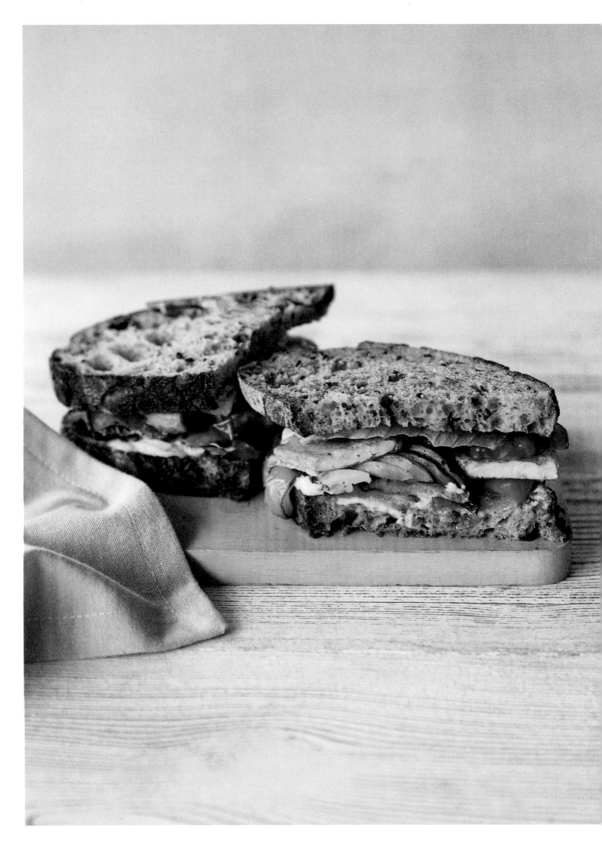

VEGAN TOFU AND VEGGIE SANDWICH

SERVES 4 | **PREP:** 15 minutes | **COOK:** 20–25 minutes

This is the vegan answer to a BLT but made with tofu, lettuce, tomato and roasted vegetables. Tofu is a good source of plant protein as it contains all eight essential amino acids as well as calcium, iron, magnesium, zinc, copper and phosphorus– most of the bone-strengthening minerals. Pan-frying it in a little oil until it's golden and crisp adds texture and flavour.

1 red or yellow pepper, deseeded and cut into 4 pieces

1 red onion, quartered

1 small aubergine, sliced into rounds

4 tbsp olive oil

400g (14oz) extra-firm tofu

2 tbsp cornflour

2 tbsp sunflower oil

8 slices wholegrain or multiseed bread

4 tbsp vegan mayonnaise

1 ripe tomato, thinly sliced

hot sauce, such as Sriracha, for drizzling (optional)

a few crisp cos or iceberg lettuce leaves

salt and freshly ground black pepper

....

Tip: Coating the tofu with cornflour before frying makes them crispy and prevents them sticking to the pan.

....

Variations:

- Use mashed avocado or vegan cream cheese instead of vegan mayo.
- Vary the roasted vegetables: try mushrooms or courgettes

1 Preheat the oven to 220°C (200°C fan/425°F/Gas 7).

2 Put the red or yellow pepper, onion and aubergine on a baking tray and drizzle with 2 tablespoons olive oil. Season lightly with salt and pepper. Roast in the preheated oven for 20–25 minutes, or until tender.

3 Cut the tofu into slices and dust lightly with cornflour. Season with salt and pepper. Heat the remaining oil in a frying pan over a medium heat and cook the tofu, in batches (do not overcrowd the pan), for 1–2 minutes each side until crisp and golden. Remove with a slotted spoon and drain on kitchen paper.

4 Lightly toast the bread and spread 4 slices with the vegan mayonnaise. Arrange the roasted vegetables over the other 4 slices and top with the hot fried tofu and sliced tomato. Drizzle with hot sauce (if using) and cover with lettuce. Top with the remaining toasted bread and cut the sandwiches in half or into quarters. Serve immediately.

FRUIT AND NUT POWER BARS

MAKES 12 | **PREP:** 15 minutes | **COOK:** 30 minutes

These gluten-free crunchy bars give you a nutritional boost when you're hungry and don't have time for a sit-down meal. The dried fruit and honey provide sweetness while the porridge oats are low GI (glycaemic index), releasing energy slowly into your bloodstream to keep you going.

1 tbsp pumpkin seeds

1 tbsp sunflower seeds

1 tbsp sesame seeds

1 tbsp chia seeds

300g (10oz) porridge oats

85g (3oz) walnuts, chopped

85g (3oz) ready-to-eat dried apricots, chopped

85g (3oz) stoned Medjool dates, chopped

85g (3oz) raisins

60g (2oz) dried cranberries

150g (5½oz) butter, plus extra for greasing

6 tbsp clear honey

Tip: If you feel indulgent, add some dark chocolate chips (70% minimum cocoa solids) to the mixture or drizzle with melted dark chocolate.

Variations:

• Use chopped pecans, hazelnuts or almonds instead of walnuts.

• Experiment with prunes, dried figs, cherries, blueberries and sultanas.

• Try different seeds: hemp, linseed or poppy seeds.

1 Preheat the oven to 160°C (140°C fan/325°F/Gas 3). Lightly butter a shallow rectangular 30 x 20cm (12 x 8in) baking tin and line with baking parchment.

2 Put the seeds in a small bowl and mix together. Put the oats, walnuts and dried fruit in a large mixing bowl.

3 Stir the butter and honey in a small pan set over a low heat until the butter melts. Add to the oat mixture and stir well. Add the seeds and mix thoroughly. If it's too dry, add a little more melted butter; if it's too sticky, add some more oats.

4 Spoon the mixture into the lined baking tin and level the top, pressing down firmly with the back of a metal spoon. Bake in the preheated oven for 30 minutes or until golden brown and starting to crisp.

5 Remove and allow to cool slightly in the tin before cutting into 12 bars. Leave until completely cold, then remove from the tin and store in an airtight container for up to 5 days.

HIGH-ENERGY SNACK BALLS

MAKES approx. 30 | **PREP:** 15 minutes | **CHILL:** 1–2 hours

Not only delicious but also nutrient dense, these bite-sized energy balls provide protein, zinc, copper, iron, magnesium and phosphorus. They can be stored in the fridge or freezer for up to three months. Vegans can use agave or maple syrup instead of honey.

175g (6oz) peanut butter (no added sugar)

90ml (3fl oz) clear honey

175g (6oz) rolled porridge oats

30g (1oz) flax seeds or chia seeds

30g (1oz) dried blueberries

60g (2oz) dark chocolate chips (minimum 70% cocoa solids)

30g (1oz) shredded unsweetened coconut

....

Tip: You can use a microwave to blend the peanut butter and honey.

....

Variations:

- Roll the balls in porridge oats or finely chopped walnuts.
- Substitute almond or cashew butter for the peanut butter.
- Blitz some dates to a sticky paste and substitute for some of the nut butter.

1 Put the peanut butter and honey in a saucepan over a low heat and stir gently until just warm (not too hot) and well blended.

2 Remove from the heat and stir in the oats, seeds, blueberries and chocolate chips, distributing them evenly throughout the mixture. If it's too sticky, add some more oats; too dry, moisten with a little cold water.

3 Take small spoonfuls of the mixture and, with your hands, mould them into small balls. Roll them in the coconut until they are sparsely coated all over.

4 Place the balls on a large cookie sheet lined with parchment paper and chill in the fridge for 1–2 hours until set firm. Transfer to an airtight container and store in the fridge for up to 10 days.

PARMESAN ROASTED ALMONDS

SERVES 8 | **PREP:** 5 minutes | **COOK:** 10–15 minutes

These fragrant roasted almonds contain a jackpot of healthy bone-strengthening nutrients, including protein, vitamin D, calcium, magnesium, phosphorus, potassium, iron, copper and zinc. You can substitute other nuts, including cashews and walnuts, or try mixing them together for variety.

3 tbsp clear honey

1 tbsp olive oil

4 tbsp grated Parmesan cheese

1 tsp smoked paprika

½ tsp chilli powder

1 tsp garlic powder

300g (10oz) whole almonds

1 tsp fine sea salt flakes

Tip: Keep an eye on the almonds while they are baking to make sure they do not get too brown or burn.

Variations:

• Vary the spices: try ground cumin, sweet paprika and cayenne.

• Add a good pinch of dried oregano, thyme or rosemary.

• For a less sweet and healthier option, use a beaten egg white instead of honey and oil. Bake the almonds for 15-20 minutes.

1 Preheat the oven to 190°C (170°C fan/375°F/Gas 5). Line a baking tray with parchment paper.

2 In a large bowl, mix together the honey, oil, Parmesan, ground spices and garlic powder. Stir in the almonds, mixing until they are evenly coated.

3 Spread the almonds out in a single layer on the lined baking tray. Sprinkle the sea salt over the top.

4 Bake in the preheated oven, turning the almonds once every 3–5 minutes, for 10–15 minutes until golden brown all over.

5 Remove from the oven and set aside to cool on the baking tray. When they are cold, store in an airtight container for up to 1 week.

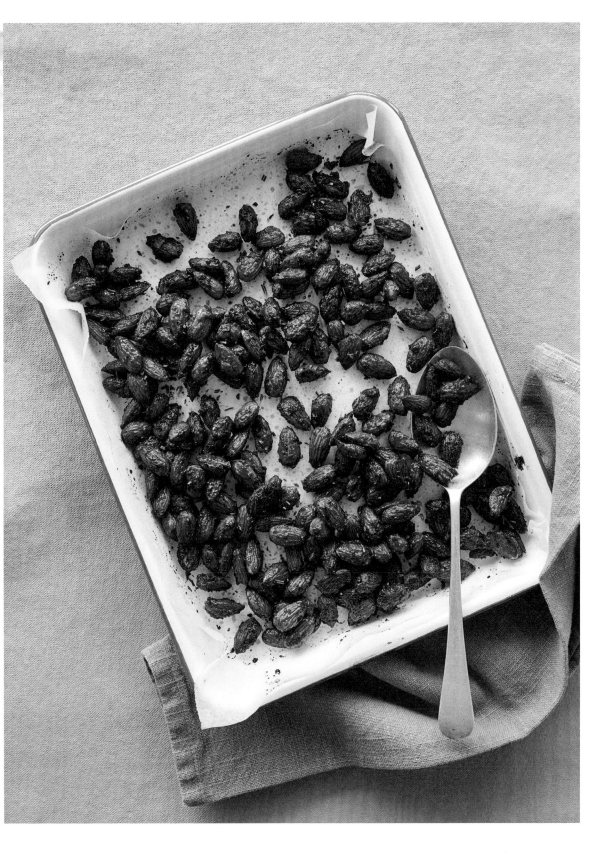

Although we know much about the incredibly complex processes related to bone, and that a delicate balance of nutrients is integral to bone health, there is still much we don't know.

The nature of science is that it is always moving forwards and, as new technological methods are developed for studying bones, we will learn more about how to maintain them. When advice is formulated for any public health matter, the caveat is always that this is the best advice given what we know at the time – there may well be knowledge gaps that we fill in the future that change these recommendations.

We have little control over some things that affect bones: taking medication for an illness, for example, may be unavoidable, and the benefits may far outweigh the risks to bone health. Lifestyle factors such as shift work may also be out of our control. There are plenty of factors that we can control, however, to ensure optimum bone health. It is important to note that just implementing one change, such as taking a vitamin D supplement, is unlikely to have a large effect on its own, but by taking a holistic approach that involves a number of positive diet and lifestyle changes can significantly improve our bone health. Here are nine key recommendations that you should practise to ensure good bone health throughout your life.

By taking a holistic approach that involves a number of positive diet and lifestyle changes, we can significantly improve our bone health.

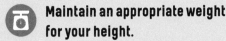 **Maintain an appropriate weight for your height.**
A good way to determine this is to calculate your body mass index (BMI) and see if it falls within the healthy zone (*see page 23*). There are also online BMI calculators.

Eat a balanced and varied diet containing plenty of plant-based foods.
Eating plenty of fruit, vegetables, wholegrain carbohydrates (such as brown rice), protein and some fat will ensure you supply your body with the correct range of vitamins, minerals and phytonutrients.

Manage internal inflammation.
Some foods, such as refined sugars, cause inflammation in the body which can affect bone health. Following a diet like the Mediterranean diet (*see page 78*), will give you everything you need without too much of what you don't, ensuring inflammation is kept to a minimum.

Get enough sleep.
Bone-building cells are linked to our circadian cycle and need us to sleep well and at the right times in order to function effectively. Seek advice from your GP if you have persistent sleep problems.

 If you don't get a lot of sun, take a vitamin D supplement.
This is important if you have dark skin, cover your skin or spend most of your time inside, even in the summer.

 Do regular weight-bearing exercise.
This type of exercise strengthens bone and encourages bone regeneration. Combining weight-bearing exercise with activities that involve impact and balance brings even greater benefits.

 Take steps to reduce stress in your life.
Reducing cortisol levels is important for bone health. Try practising meditation or mindfulness to alleviate stress and seek medical help if you find you cannot manage your stress levels.

 Give up smoking.
This will benefit your whole body, not just your bones.

Limit alcohol intake to under 14 units week.
Alcohol in moderate amounts is unlikely to harm bones, but excessive intake can affect bone density.

BIBLIOGRAPHY

INTRODUCTION

[1] Dyer, S.M., Crotty, M., Fairhall, N., et al. 'A critical review of the long-term disability outcomes following hip fracture.' *BMC Geriatrics* (2016); 16:158.

THE SCIENCE

[1 and 2] Mohamad, N.V., Soelaiman, I.N., Chin, K.Y. 'A concise review of testosterone and bone health.' *Clinical Interventions in Aging* (2016); 11:1317–24.

[3] Sansone, R.A., Sansone, L.A. 'SSRIs: bad to the bone?' *Innovations in Clinical Neuroscience* (2012); 9(7–8):42–47.

[4] Cohen, A., Dempster, D.W., Recker, R.R., Lappe, J.M., Zhou, H., Zwahlen, A., Müller, R., Zhao, B., Guom, X., Lang, T., Saeed, I., et al. 'Abdominal fat is associated with lower bone formation and inferior bone quality in healthy premenopausal women: a transiliac bone biopsy study.' *The Journal of Clinical Endocrinology and Metabolism* (2013); 98:6:2562–72.

[5] Shapses, S.A., Pop, L.C., Wang, Y. 'Obesity is a concern for bone health with aging.' *Nutritional Research* (2017); 39:1–13.

[6] Park, H.A., Lee, J. S., Kuller, L.H., Cauley, J.A. 'Effects of weight control during the menopausal transition on bone mineral density.' *The Journal of Clinical Endocrinology and Metabolism* (2007); 92:10:3809–15.

[7] Rothschild, D., Weissbrod, O., Barkan, E., Kurilshikov, A., Korem, T., Zeevi, D., Costea, P.I., Godneva, A., Kalka, I.N., Bar, N., Shilo, S., Lador, D., et al. 'Environment dominates over host genetics in shaping human gut microbiota.' *Nature* (2018); 555:210–15.

[8] LaBrie, J.W., Boyle, S., Earle, A., Almstedt, H.C. 'Heavy episodic drinking is associated with poorer bone health in adolescent and young adult women.' *J Stud Alcohol Drugs* (2018); 79(3):391–98.

[9] Swanson, C.M., Kohrt, W.M., Buxton, O.M., Everson, C.A., Wright, K.P., Jr, Orwoll, E.S., Shea, S.A. 'The importance of the circadian system and sleep for bone health.' *Metabolism* (2018); 84:28–43.

EXERCISE

[1] Phillips, C., Fahimi, A. 'Immune and neuroprotective effects of physical activity on the brain in depression.' *Frontiers In Neuroscience* (2018); 12:498.

[2] Aluoch, A.O., Jessee, R., Habal, H., Garcia-Rosell, M., Shah, R., Reed, G., Carbone, L. 'Heart failure as a risk factor for osteoporosis and fractures.' *Current Osteoporosis Report* (2012); 10(4):258–69.

NUTRITION

[1] Whisner, C.M., Castillo, L.F. 'Prebiotics, bone and mineral metabolism.' *Calcified Tissue International* (2018); 102(4):443–79.

[2] Brot, C., Darsø, P. 'The Danish Health and Medicines Authority recommendations regarding prevention, diagnosis and treatment of vitamin D deficiency.' *Rational Pharmacotherapy* (2010); 6.

[3] Lips, P., Cashman, K., Lamberg-Allardt, C., Bischoff-Ferrari, H., Obermayer-Pietsch, B., Bianchi, M., Stepan, J., El-Hajj Fuleihan, G., Bouillon, R. 'Current vitamin D status in European and Middle East countries and strategies to prevent vitamin D deficiency: a position statement of the European Calcified Tissue Society.' *European Journal of Endocrinology* (2019); 180(4):23–54.

[4] Allen, L., de Benoist, B., Dary, O., Hurrell, R. (eds). 'Guidelines on food fortification with micronutrients.' *World Health Organization* (2016). www.who.int/nutrition/publications/guide_food_fortification_micronutrients.pdf

[5] 'Vegetables – food supply quantity.' *Food and Agricultural Organization of the United Nations* (2020). www.fao.org/faostat/en/#data/FBS

[6] 'Say hello to a fortified future: 2016 year in review.' *Food Fortification Initiative* (2016). http://ffinetwork.org/about/stay_informed/publications/documents/FFI2016Review.pdf

[7] DiNicolantonio, J.J., Mehta, V., Zaman, S.B., O'Keefe, J.H. 'Not salt but sugar as aetiological in osteoporosis: a review.' *Missouri State Medical Association* (2018); 115(3):247–52.

[8] Wikoff, D., Welsh, B.T., Henderson, R., et al. 'Systematic review of the potential adverse effects of caffeine consumption in healthy adults, pregnant women, adolescents and children.' *Food and Chemical Toxicology* (2017); 109(Pt 1):585–648.

INDEX

AUTHOR ACKNOWLEDGEMENTS

I would like to thank Victoria Marshallsay for first attending one of my talks and then remembering me afterwards, and Lisa Dyer for her confidence and reassurance towards the end. I would also like to thank Olly Figg for being my mentor and always on hand for advice, and my husband Tom for being my cheerleader.

Thanks to Heather Thomas for her mouth-watering recipes and Bianca Sainty for converting the science into practical and achievable exercises.

And not least to the countless researchers whose findings allow us a window into the fascinating and complex workings of our bodies.

Jo Travers

ABOUT THE CONTRIBUTORS

Bianca Sainty is a London-based Personal Trainer and the founder of Pod Fitness — specialists in outdoor small-group personal training. A former TV producer, Bianca retrained in 2013 to gain an Advanced Diploma in Personal Training from YMCAFit. More recently she has added the FitPro Live Osteoporosis Workshop and Exercise for Older Adults to her qualifications. You can exercise with Bianca on her YouTube channel "Workout with B" or connect with her on Instagram @biancasainty.

Heather Thomas is a food writer and editor and the author of several bestselling health and cookery books, including *The Avocado Cookbook* and *The Greek Vegetarian Cookbook*. She has worked with many top chefs, nutritionists and women's health organizations and charities.

PICTURE CREDITS

Shutterstock, Inc: 4L, 8 Xray Computer; 10 NastyaSigne; 11 Alexander_P; 12, 32 elenabsl; 13 Arisa_J; 15 VectorMine; 16 naulicrea; 17, 35 Double Brain; 18 Designua; 21 Andrii Bezershenko; 21BR PeoGeo; 22, 23TR, 25L, 26R, 28 Rahib Valiyev; 24T vectorchef; 24B Sulee_R; 25R Art studio G; 26L NirdalArt; 30 Neokryuger; 4R, 36 Goran Bogicevic; 39 ESB Professional; 43 Iryna Inshyna; 44, 48, 50, 51 F8 studio; 45 fizkes; 46 Tatyana Chaiko; 47 Ansoul; 49 Mihai Blanaru; 52 ruigsantos; 53 Kotin; 5L, 54 Alexandra Anschiz; 56 Natalia Lisovskaya; 58 nadianb; 59 New Africa; 61 Ekaterina Markelova; 62 yanikap; 63 Eva Gruendemann; 65 Veliavik; 67 Subbotina Anna; 68 luchschenF; 69 ch_ch; 71 Svetlana Lukienko; 72T Liliya Kandrashevich; 72B tarapong srichaiyos; 73 mangkenark; 74 Elena Hramova; 76T alesjab; 76B Fascinadora; 77 Evgeny Karandaev; 78 Foxys Forest Manufacture; 81 Nina Firsova. © **Welbeck Non-Fiction Limited:** 21, 23BL, 35, 40. **Izy Hossack** © **Welbeck Non-Fiction Limited:** 5R, 82–121.

Senior Commissioning Editor: Victoria Marshallsay   **Designer:** Louise Evans
Photographer: Izy Hossack   **Food and Props Stylist:** Dominique Eloise Alexander
Copy Editor: Anna Cheifetz   **Proofreader:** Jane Birch   **Indexer:** Angie Hipkin
Production Controller: Gary Hayes